Anticoagulation Drugs - the Current State of the Art

Edited by Mina Kelleni

Published in London, United Kingdom

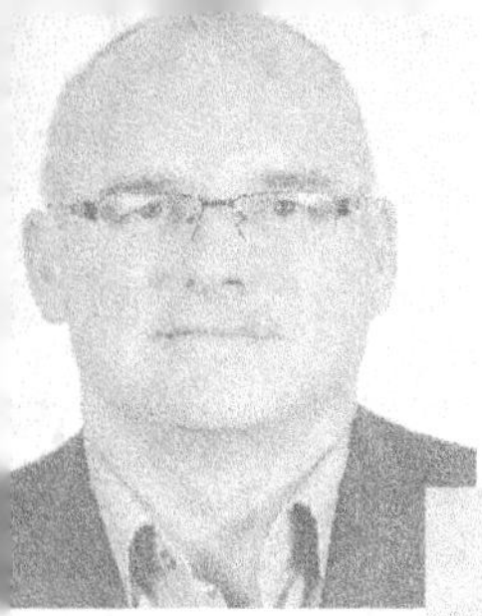
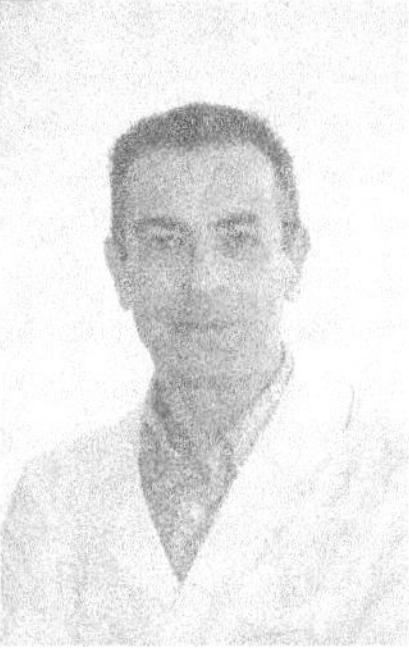
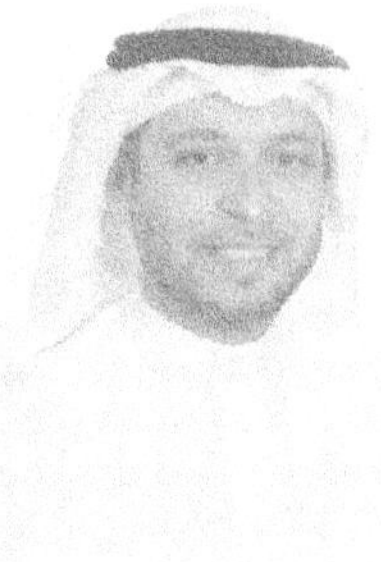
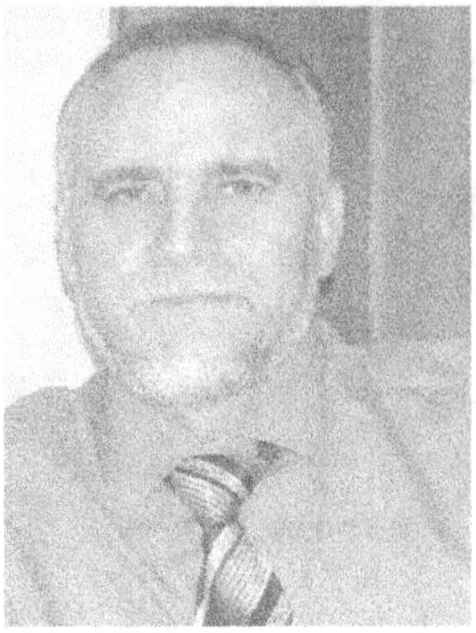
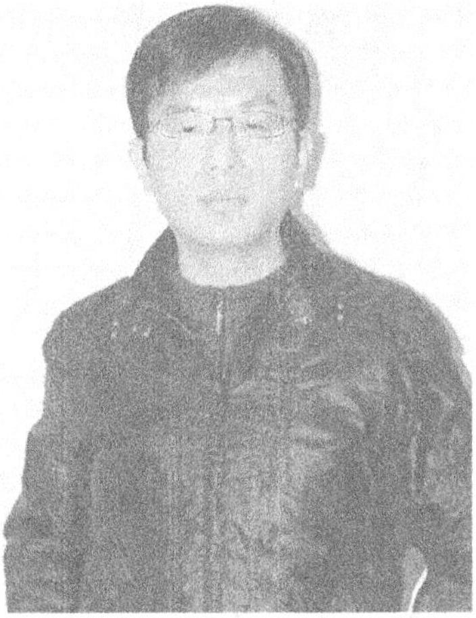
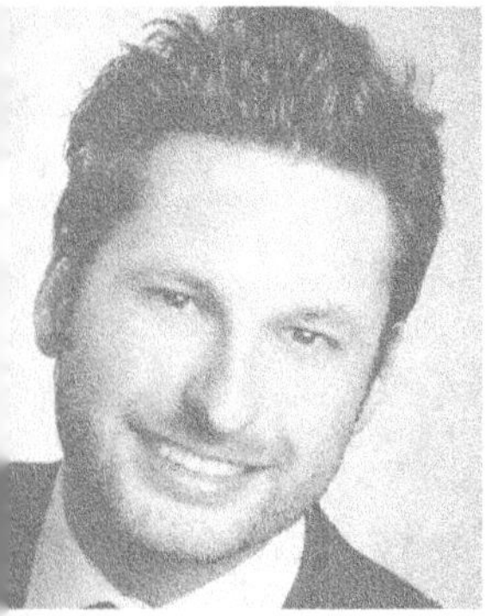
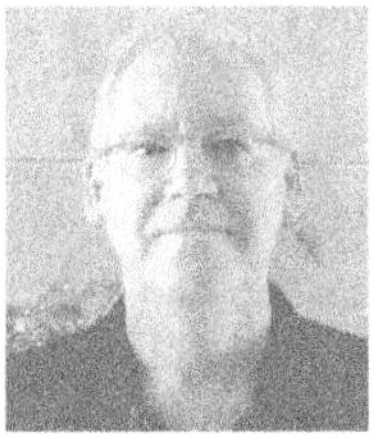

IntechOpen

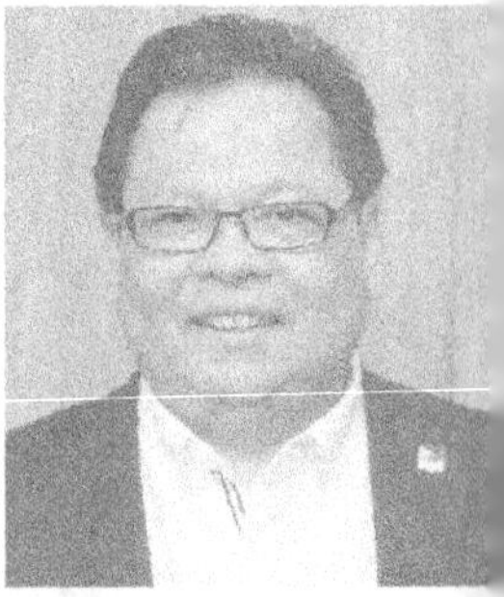
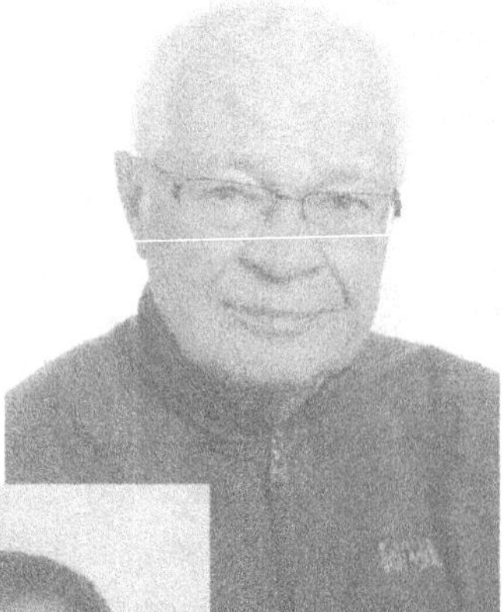
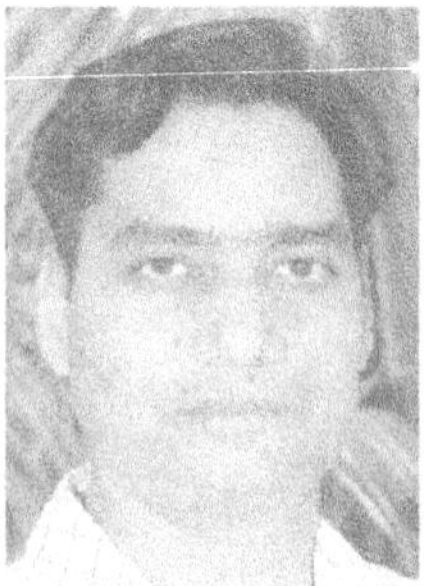
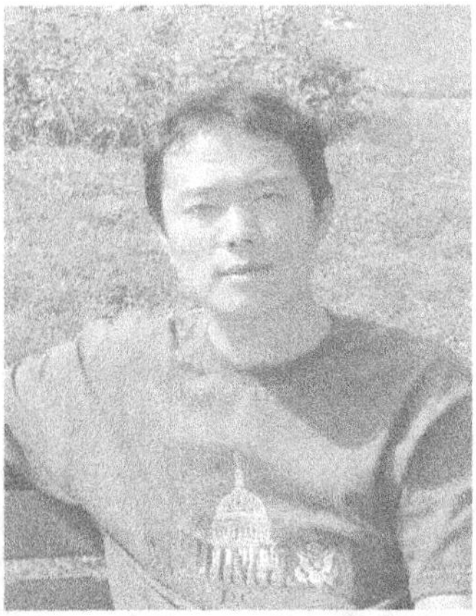
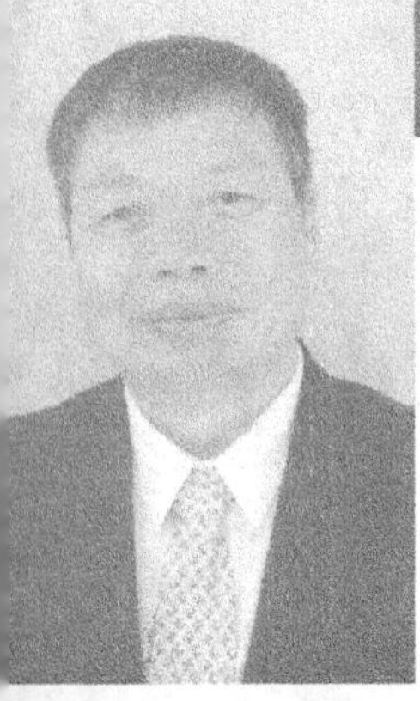
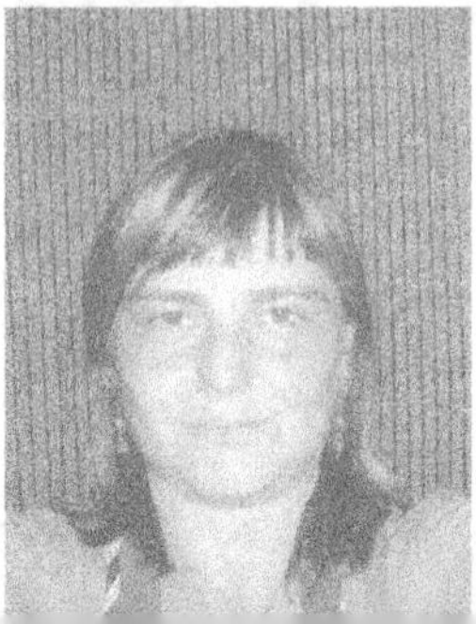

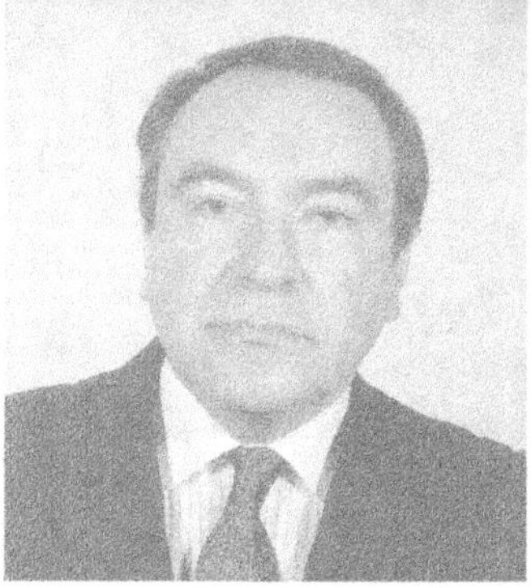

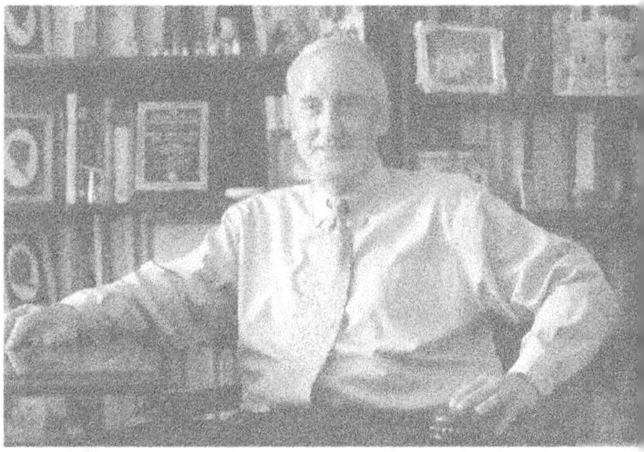

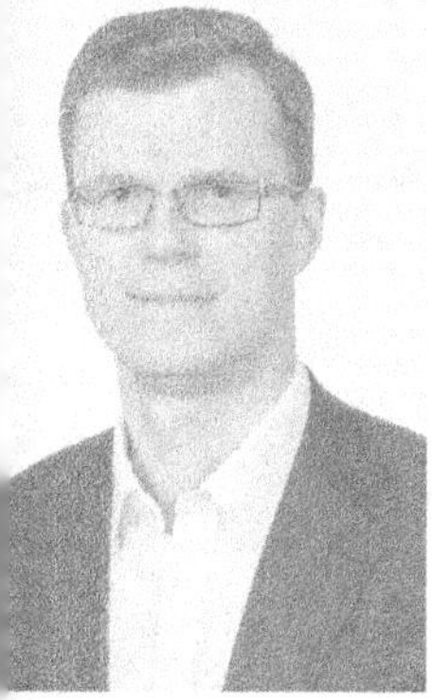

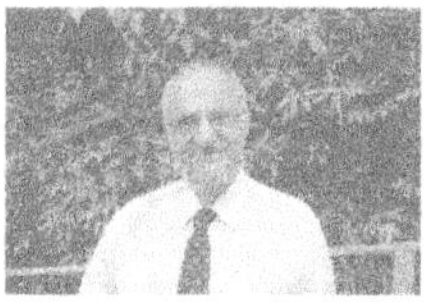

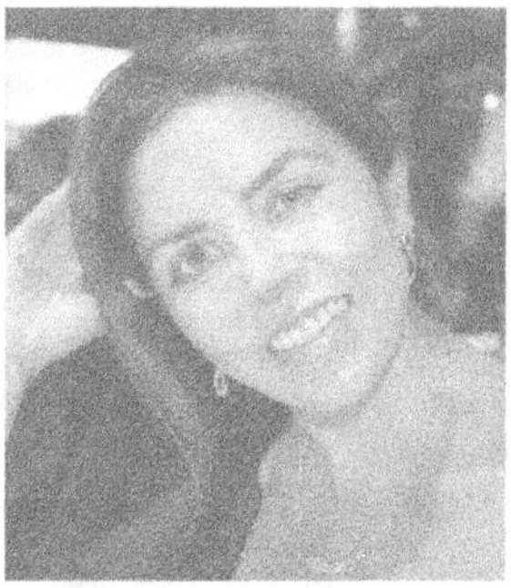

Supporting open minds since 2005

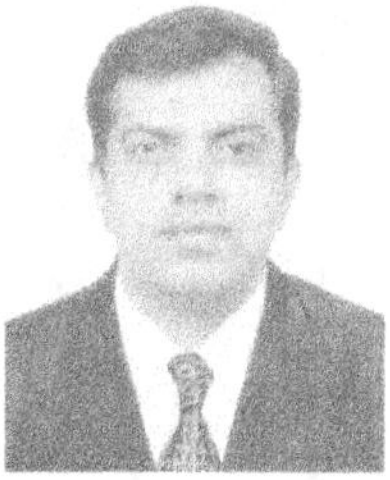

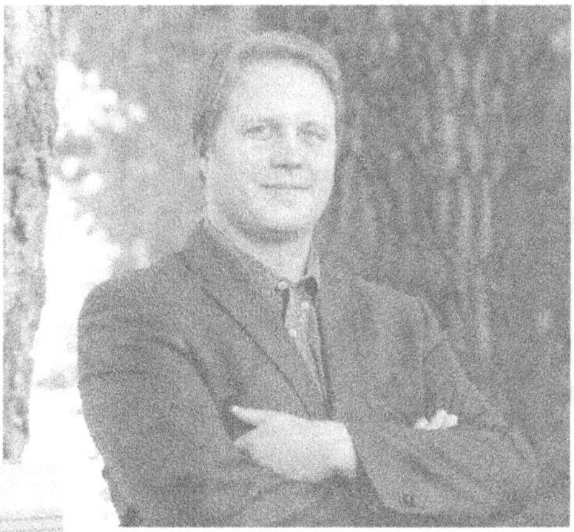

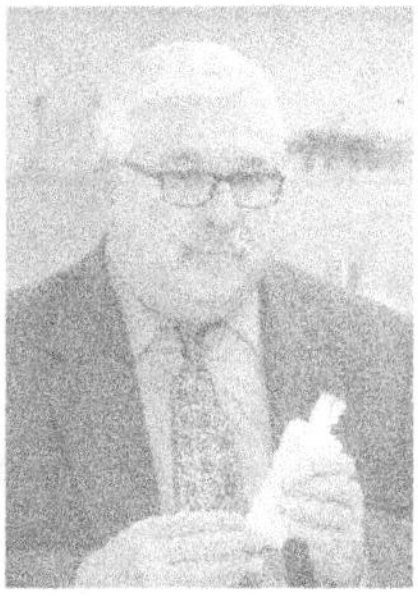

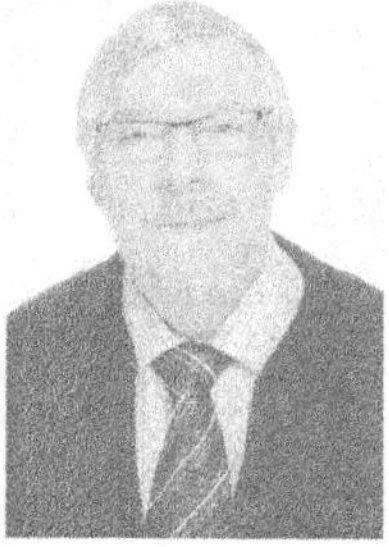

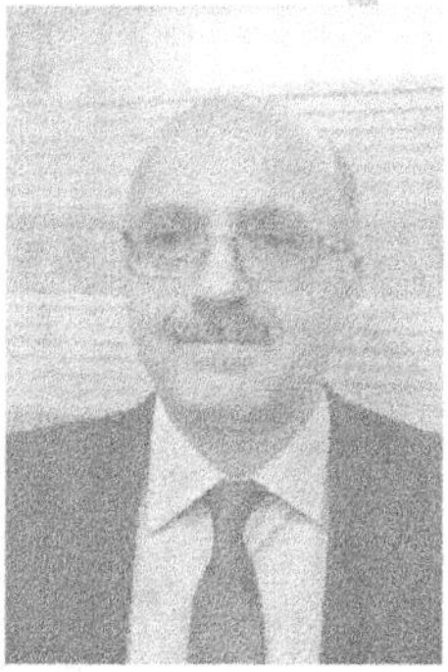

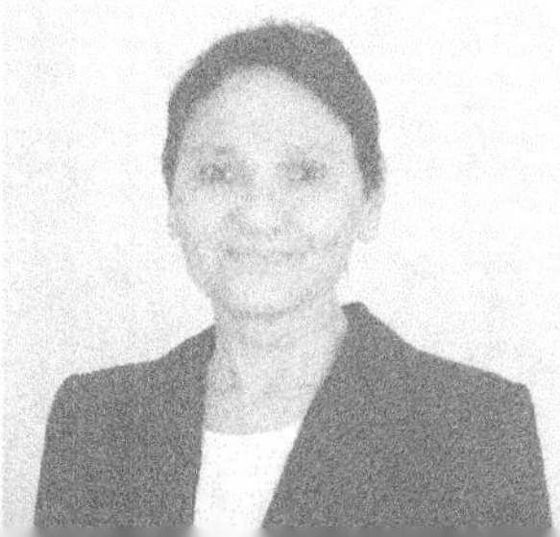

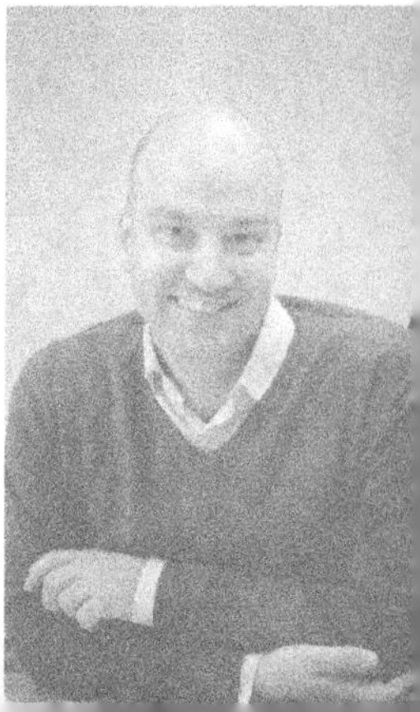

Anticoagulation Drugs - the Current State of the Art
http://dx.doi.org/10.5772/intechopen.80117
Edited by Mina Kelleni

Contributors
Jean Amiral, Anne Marie Vissac, Yetti Hernaningsih, Ersa Bayung Maulidan, Hobart Owen Ng Tsai, Dr. Laila Matalqah, Mina T. Kelleni

First published in London, United Kingdom, 2020 by IntechOpen
IntechOpen is the global imprint of INTECHOPEN LIMITED, registered in England and Wales, registration number: 11086078, 7th floor, 10 Lower Thames Street, London, EC3R 6AF, United Kingdom
Printed in Croatia

British Library Cataloguing-in-Publication Data
A catalogue record for this book is available from the British Library

Additional hard and PDF copies can be obtained from orders@intechopen.com

Anticoagulation Drugs - the Current State of the Art
Edited by Mina Kelleni
p. cm.
Print ISBN 978-1-78985-075-8
Online ISBN 978-1-78985-076-5
eBook (PDF) ISBN 978-1-83880-145-8

Meet the editor

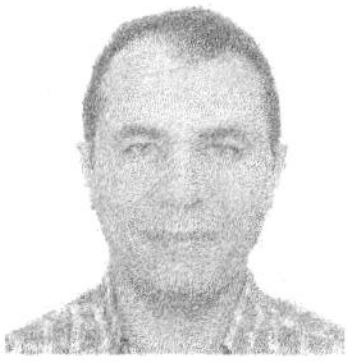

Dr Mina Kelleni graduated from the College of Medicine, Minia University, Egypt and chose a career in pharmacology, which became the passion of his life and clinical research. He currently works as an assistant professor of pharmacology at both the Faculty of Medicine, Minia University, Egypt as well as the College of Pharmacy, Jouf University, KSA. Dr Kelleni has been acting as an editorial board member of numerous international medical journals in several fields of medicine and endocrinology, and he has been invited as a speaker to more than 100 international medical conferences all over the globe. Recently, Dr Kelleni has also filed for registration of two patents involving new drugs dealing with epilepsy and premature ejaculation.

Contents

Preface

Hemorrhage is one of the nightmare conditions that every physician will experience regardless of the specialty he chose. Some physicians encounter hemorrhages on a daily basis such as ER doctors, and others less frequently and sometimes rarely. A basic knowledge for the calm specialties and an advanced one for the troublesome are highly required. Once I was contacted by IntechOpen to edit this book on anticoagulants, I accepted immediately. I hope that the reader may find both basic and advanced knowledge about this highly important group of drugs In every chapter of "Anticoagulation Drugs - the Latest Developments" you'll find both basic and advanced knowledge to help the beginners in the field as well as to satisfy the experts. I'm very grateful to Mrs. Nina Kalinic Babic, the author service manager, who has provided relentless and highly professional support through every step during preparation and editing of this book. Finally, I would like to appreciate the joy and support provided by my lovely family; Ereny, Elena, and Eleanor to whom I owe my life.

Mina T. Kelleni, MD, PhD
Minia University,
Egypt

College of Pharmacy,
Jouf University,
KSA

Section 1

Introduction

Chapter 1

Introductory Chapter: Anticoagulant Therapy in Clinical Practice - Challenges and Wishes

Mina T. Kelleni

1. Introduction

Since the discovery of heparin in 1915, anticoagulant drugs have played a vital role in prophylaxis of deep vein thrombosis and pulmonary thromboembolism among other important indications, and for more than six decades, both heparin and coumarins especially warfarin have been the principal drugs used for anticoagulation worldwide [1, 2]. In the mid-1970s and the 1980s, several low-molecular-weight heparins have been clinically trialed and commercialized, and over the past few decades, parenteral direct thrombin inhibitors (DTIs) (e.g., argatroban, bivalirudin), oral DTIs (e.g., dabigatran), and oral direct factor Xa inhibitors (e.g., rivaroxaban) have also been introduced into the clinical practice to cope with the growing use of anticoagulants in medicine [1, 3, 4].

The clinical practice involving the use of anticoagulants, e.g., dosing, timing, and managing complications, has been a real challenge even to some of the best experts in the field mainly due to their potential to cause serious adverse effects, both hemorrhagic and nonhemorrhagic which may occur with all the currently used anticoagulants regardless of their year of discovery [2, 5–8].

Thus, in this book you'll find experts' opinion providing state-of-art knowledge regarding current clinical usage and monitoring of anticoagulant therapy. It discusses some very critical subjects like the mechanism and heterogenic presentation of heparin-induced thrombocytopenia, laboratory monitoring of heparin anticoagulants, quality of life among patients, as well as an updated pharmacological review of the currently used anticoagulants and their antidotes. Our main aim is to improve the clinical practice of all physicians and healthcare providers who are dealing with anticoagulants as well as to present an added value to the current literature discussing the complications experienced while using anticoagulants. We're still waiting for the synthesis of an ideal or almost ideal anticoagulant which combines both efficacy and lack of serious adverse effects [9].

Author details

Mina T. Kelleni[1,2]

1 Faculty of Medicine, Minia University, Egypt

2 College of Pharmacy, Jouf University, KSA

*Address all correspondence to: mina.kelleni@mu.edu.eg

References

[1] Gomez-Outes A, Suarez-Gea ML, Calvo-Rojas G, et al. Discovery of anticoagulant drugs: A historical perspective. Current Drug Discovery Technologies. 2012;**9**(2):83-104

[2] Gallerani M, Manfredini R, Moratelli S. Non-haemorrhagic adverse reactions of oral anticoagulant therapy. International Journal of Cardiology. 1995;**49**(1):1-7

[3] Torri G, Naggi A. Heparin centenary—An ever-young life-saving drug. International Journal of Cardiology. 2016;**212**(Suppl 1):S1-S4

[4] Le Pogam MA, Quantin C, Reich O, et al. Geriatric patient safety indicators based on linked administrative health data to assess anticoagulant-related thromboembolic and hemorrhagic adverse events in older inpatients: A study proposal. JMIR Research Protocols. 2017;**6**(5):e82

[5] Alshammari TM, Ata SI, Mahmoud MA, Alhawassi TM, Aljadhey HS. Signals of bleeding among direct-acting oral anticoagulant users compared to those among warfarin users: Analyses of the post-marketing FDA adverse event reporting system (FAERS) database, 2010-2015. Therapeutics and Clinical Risk Management. 2018;**14**:803-809

[6] Eek AK, Strom BO, Bakkehoi G, Stenberg-Nilsen H. Anticoagulant-associated adverse drug reactions in 2013-15. Tidsskrift for den Norske Lægeforening. 2018;**138**(12):1-11

[7] Leong WA. Case studies in anticoagulation management. Journal of Thrombosis and Thrombolysis. 2008;**25**(1):78-84

[8] Liu Z, Han N, Xu H, et al. Incidence of venous thromboembolism and hemorrhage related safety studies of preoperative anticoagulation therapy in hip fracture patients undergoing surgical treatment: A case-control study. BMC Musculoskeletal Disorders. 2016;**17**:76

[9] Haas S. New anticoagulants—Towards the development of an "ideal" anticoagulant. VASA. 2009;**38**(1):13-29

Section 2

Current Anticoagulation Therapy: Practice and Monitoring

Chapter 2

Pharmacological Review of Anticoagulants

Hobart Owen Ng Tsai

Abstract

The art and science of anticoagulation have never gotten more complicated than it has now. Newer anticoagulants have entered the market and have provided more options to the patients and healthcare professionals. This chapter will review the basic physiology of hemostasis, pharmacology of the anticoagulants, and how these medications are used in the clinical setting. The mechanism of action, pharmacokinetics and pharmacodynamics, clinical evidence of use and clinical pearls, laboratory monitoring in clinical practice, and adverse effects will be examined individually for each drug considered. This chapter will serve as a review for the practicing clinician and a thorough introduction for the beginning reader.

Keywords: anticoagulants, warfarin, heparin, low molecular weight heparin, enoxaparin, dabigatran, rivaroxaban, apixaban, edoxaban

1. Introduction

Anticoagulants are the mainstay of treatment for stroke and systemic embolism prevention in patients with atrial fibrillation (AF) or flutter. They can be used as well for prevention and treatment of venous thromboembolism (VTE) and treatment of thrombus formation in other places. This class of medications must be used carefully because using them incorrectly can lead to either ineffective prevention of clot formation or bleeding. It is vital for the clinician who uses any of these anticoagulants to have a basic understanding of their pharmacology and evidence of use.

2. The coagulation cascade

The coagulation system is composed of two separate pathways that convene on a single pathway. The two pathways are extrinsic pathway and intrinsic pathway. Injury to the endothelial system exposes *tissue factor* out in the bloodstream. The extrinsic pathway begins with factor VII. Circulating factor VII in the bloodstream will then get activated to factor VIIa when they come into contact with tissue factor. Factor VIIa then converts factors X and IX to factor Xa and IXa, respectively. The presence of factor IXa, together with factor VIIIa, work to produce more factor Xa. Factor Xa and factor Va then activate factor II (prothrombin) to factor IIa (thrombin). Factor IIa then converts fibrinogen to fibrin [1, 2].

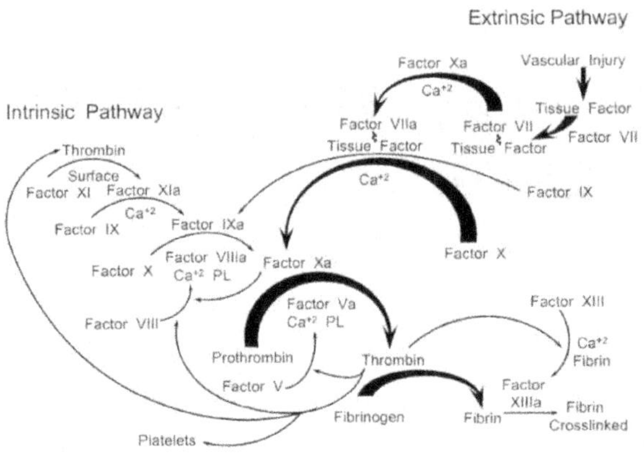

Figure 1.
Coagulation cascade showing the intrinsic, extrinsic, and common pathway. Reprint with permission from [30].

The result of this cascade is the production of fibrin molecules that bind to GPIIb/IIIa receptors on platelets and hold them together to form a platelet plug. The extrinsic pathway is what protects humans when bleeding occurs involving trauma to the vasculature or when the blood comes in contact with extravascular tissues [1, 2].

The intrinsic pathway gets activated upon trauma to the blood or when the blood gets exposed to collagen found on damaged blood vessels. At the beginning of the intrinsic pathway activation, exposure of factor XII to collagen, for example, stimulates a configurational change in factor XII to become factor XIIa. Together the help of high molecular weight kininogen and prekallikrein, factor XIIa enzymatically activates factor XI to XIa. Factor XIa in turn activates factor IX to IXa. Factor IXa then works with factor VIIIa to convert factor X to Xa. Factor Xa then converts factor II to factor IIa, which in turn activates fibrinogen to fibrin [1, 2].

The extrinsic pathway and intrinsic pathway converge as the common pathway when factor X gets converted to factor Xa [1, 2] (see **Figure 1**).

3. Basic and clinical pharmacology of the anticoagulants

3.1 Unfractionated heparin (UFH)

3.1.1 Mechanism of action

Unfractionated heparin is a long string of glycosaminoglycan molecules that can range from 3000 to 30,000 Daltons. UFH with its specific pentasaccharide sequence binds to antithrombin III and catalyzes its efficiency in inhibiting factor Xa and IIa in a ratio of 1: 1. However, not all heparin molecules given are active; only about a third of the heparin molecules in a solution contain the required pentasaccharide sequence [1–3].

3.1.2 ADME

Heparin is not absorbed orally and is given either subcutaneously (SQ) or intravenously (IV). Heparin is highly protein bound and is cleared in the bloodstream by endothelial cells and macrophages. The half-life of heparin increases as the dose increases; it can vary from 1 hour at a dose of 100 units/kg to 2.5 h for 400 units/kg to 5 h for 800 units/kg. In general, the clinical effect of IV UFH dissipates 4–6 hours after stopping the infusion [1–3].

3.1.3 Clinical use

UFH can be either given SQ or IV as mentioned above. However, SQ administration of UFH has erratic bioavailability. Hence, SQ is not a preferred route if a patient requires treatment dose of UFH. Clinical studies have also shown a higher rate of treatment failure rate with SQ compared to IV heparin [3, 4]. For VTE prophylaxis, SQ administration of UFH would suffice. The usual dose is 5000 units q8-12h [4].

Initial dosing of IV UFH depends on the indication. Besides VTE treatment, IV UFH can also be used for patients with acute coronary syndrome, as a bridging agent for patients with atrial fibrillation, mechanical valves, etc. The dose of IV UFH could be either a fixed dose or a weight-based dose. A study by Raschke et al. [3] compared fixed dose vs. weight-based dose of IV heparin in patients with venous and arterial thromboembolism. In that study, significantly more patients (97%) in the weight-based dosing group achieved an Activated Partial Thromboplastin Time (aPTT) > 1.5x the baseline within 24 hours vs. the fixed dose group (77%), leading the authors to conclude that weight-based dosing is superior to fixed dose IV heparin [3, 4]. The 2016 Guidance for the practical management of the heparin anticoagulants in the treatment of venous thromboembolism and the 2012 American College of Chest Physicians (ACCP) Guidelines on Antithrombotic Therapy and Prevention of Thrombosis Supplement on Parenteral Anticoagulants list both fixed dose and weight-based dose for IV heparin [3].

3.1.4 Monitoring

There are two ways of monitoring the heparin activity in the body. These are the aPTT and Activated Clotting Time (ACT). The usual aPTT target for a therapeutic effect of heparin is 1.5–2x the baseline, which is equivalent to an anti-factor Xa activity of 0.3–0.7 units/ml [1, 3, 4]. The target aPTT varies based on what reagent is used to measure it. Thus, the clinician should check with the institution's laboratory for the target aPTT for patients receiving IV heparin. When using IV UFH for treating heparin or for bridging purposes, the aPTT is used. Another lab test used to monitor heparin is the ACT. ACT is available as a point-of-care test and is used when patients are receiving high doses of heparin. ACT can be seen being used in instances such as during cardiopulmonary bypass surgery and percutaneous coronary intervention. The target ACT varies based on the indication. ACT is reported in seconds and denotes how long it takes for the blood to clot.

3.1.5 Adverse effects

Patients on heparin also need close monitoring of platelet counts. Thrombocytopenia could be a consequence of heparin infusion and severe reaction called heparin-induced thrombocytopenia (HIT) may occur [1–5]. There are two kinds of heparin-induced thrombocytopenia: HIT type 1 and HIT type 2. HIT Type 1, which may also be called heparin-associated thrombocytopenia, is a benign, transient drop in platelets counts usually within the first 2–4 days after initiation of heparin infusion. Platelet counts rarely go below 100,000 [3–6]. The mechanism behind HIT type 1 is unknown but may involve dilutional effect or decreased platelet production associated with the acute illness [6].

The other more serious reaction, which is HIT type 2, involves antibody formation against heparin-platelet factor 4 complex. Heparin may bind to platelet factor-4 (PF 4), which is a cationic protein product of platelets that binds heparin and prevents heparin from binding with antithrombin. The heparin-PF4 complex is highly antigenic and induces the formation of IgG molecules against it. The IgG molecule-heparin-PF 4 complex binds to platelets and activates it, further releasing more PF4. The activated platelets with bound IgG-heparin-PF 4 complex also produce prothrombotic molecules that may cause thrombosis [3–6]. HIT type 2 can cause both arterial and venous thromboses, although venous thrombosis is more common. The activated platelets with bound IgG-heparin-PF 4 get removed from the body quickly, hence causing thrombocytopenia [6].

For the treatment of HIT, the American Society of Hematology 2018 guidelines for the management of venous thromboembolism: heparin-induced thrombocytopenia suggests use of non-heparin options such as argatroban (a direct thrombin inhibitor), fondaparinux (an ant-factor Xa inhibitor), or DOAC (specifically rivaroxaban due to most experience at a dose of 15 mg twice a day for 3 weeks if thrombosis is present, or 15 mg twice a day until the platelet counts have recovered to $\geq 150 \times 10^9$/L, then followed by 20 mg daily if there is an indication for continued anticoagulation) [7].

3.1.6 Reversibility

In the event of bleeding, heparin can be reversed with protamine sulfate. Protamine is a cationic protein from fish sperm that can bind to heparin (which is anionic) and neutralize heparin immediately [1]. 1 mg of protamine reverses approximately 100 units of heparin, with a maximum dose of 50 mg at a time. For patients who are receiving continuous IV heparin infusion, only the last 2–3 hours dose of heparin given needs to be taken into when calculating the dose for protamine. For patients who received SQ heparin, protamine has to be given as a prolonged infusion. aPTT can be used to monitor the efficacy of protamine. One needs to be careful when giving protamine as protamine itself is prothrombotic [3, 5].

3.2 Low molecular weight heparin (LMWH)

There are various preparations of LMWH available in the market. Some examples are enoxaparin, dalteparin, tinzaparin, etc. The rest of the discussion in this section will focus on enoxaparin.

3.2.1 Mechanism of action

LMWH's are shorter molecular version of UFH. They are only a third of the size of UFH. Same as UFH, LMWH bind to antithrombin and catalyzes its efficiency. But unlike UFH, the combination LMWH-antithrombin is only capable of deactivating factor Xa and very little factor IIa [1, 3, 5].

3.2.2 ADME

Enoxaparin can be either given SQ or IV depending on the indication. It is predominantly cleared renally hence dose adjustment is needed in patients with renal impairment (when Cockcroft-Gault calculated creatinine clearance is <30 ml/min). It has a half-life of 3–6 hours and reaches peak concentration 3–5 hours after SQ injection [1, 3–5].

3.2.3 Clinical use

Enoxaparin can be given as a once a day or twice daily dosing. Once daily dosing is not advisable in certain populations such as obese patients because the effect of enoxaparin would not last for 24 hours [4]. The dose varies based on the indication.

It can be used for VTE treatment and prophylaxis, arterial thromboses, bridging agent for patients with atrial fibrillation, mechanical valves, etc. It is easier to use in practice than IV heparin if full treatment dose is needed as there is no laboratory monitoring required.

3.2.4 Monitoring

The activity of LMWH is more predictable than UFH. Hence, monitoring is not needed when LMWH is given. However, its anticoagulation effects may be determined by checking the anti-factor Xa activity. Several guidelines including the 2016 Guidelines for the practical management of the heparin anticoagulants in the treatment of venous thromboembolism and the 2018 American Society of Hematology guidelines for the management of venous thromboembolism: optimal management of anticoagulation therapy do not suggest routing monitoring of anti-factor Xa activity due to uncertainties regarding its clinical utility and its cost-effectiveness [4, 8]. Additionally, there is currently no standardized method of adjusting the dose of enoxaparin based on anti-factor Xa activity [8], except for pediatric patients.

3.2.5 Adverse effects

As with any anticoagulants, bleeding is a major concern for patients receiving LMWH. Hematoma surrounding the injection site may also appear if patients rub on the injection site. In terms of major side effects, LMWH has a lower incidence of HIT type 2 compared to UFH. However, patients who have a history of HIT type 2 should best avoid LMWH if antibodies are still present.

3.2.6 Reversibility

In cases of bleeding, enoxaparin may be partially reversed with protamine if it was given within 8 hours. Protamine can only reverse 65–70% of enoxaparin at most [5]. Protamine neutralizes anti factor IIa bound to the LMWH-antithrombin complex completely but only variably to factor Xa bound to the LMWH-antithrombin complex [3, 5].

3.3 Warfarin

3.3.1 Mechanism of action

Warfarin has been used around since the early 1930s but it was not used clinically until the 1950s. Warfarin is the oldest oral anticoagulant around. Warfarin inhibits vitamin K epoxide reductase (VKOR) that leads to the decrease in production of factors II, VII, IX, and X. These factors depend on vitamin K for carboxylation in order to become active. In addition to these four factors, vitamin K also decrease the production of protein C and S, which also depend on carboxylation to become active [5, 9, 10] (See **Figure 2**).

3.3.2 ADME

Warfarin is present as a racemic mixture of two enantiomers, S-warfarin and R-warfarin. S warfarin is about three times more potent than R-warfarin. The S-warfarin is metabolized by CYP 2C9, whereas R-warfarin is metabolized by CYP 1A1, 1A2, and 3A4. Hence, any metabolic interactions involving these enzymes, especially 2C9, would affect the clinical efficacy and safety of warfarin significantly [9, 10].

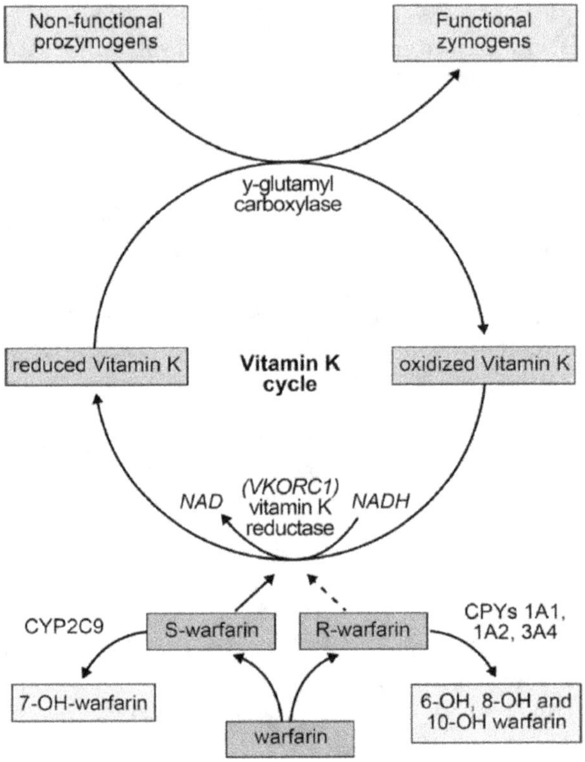

Figure 2.
Vitamin K cycle showing where warfarin acts and the enzymes that metabolize each enantiomer. Reprint with permission from [16].

Warfarin is readily absorbed and is almost 100% bioavailable. It has similar volume of distribution as albumin (0.11–0.18 L/kg) and is metabolized by the liver. It is a highly protein-bound drug (>98%) and has a half-life of 36–42 hours (R-warfarin 45 hours, S-warfarin 29 hours). Advances in genetics have elucidated that polymorphisms in the gene that encode VKOR (VKORC1) and CYP2C9 enzyme dramatically affect the dose requirement of a patient [9, 10]. Dose calculators based on the genetic polymorphisms of these two enzymes exist and some of them are available online. How accurate they are is still a question. It should be noted that each patient's warfarin dose requirement does not rely only on genes. Genetics can only account for 30–50% of each patient's dose requirement. Diet, medical condition, and drugs (including supplements) have a role to play as well in determining how much warfarin one needs.

3.3.3 Clinical use

Clinically, warfarin is used for various conditions such as prevention of stroke and systemic embolism in patients with atrial fibrillation or atrial flutter, treatment and prevention of venous thromboembolism, cerebral venous thrombosis, etc. Clinicians have the most experience with warfarin and warfarin has a wider range of indications than the direct-acting oral anticoagulants (DOACs).

There are several published sample algorithms on initiation and dosing of warfarin. Several institutions also have in-house protocols and dose adjustment guidelines for patients on warfarin. However, due to the multiple factors that can affect warfarin, the protocols may not be necessarily apt to follow. Picking the correct warfarin dose to start patients on and adjusting of warfarin doses subsequently is usually not as simple clinically. Choosing what dose to start patients on require a thorough review of that patient's medical condition, weighing thrombotic risk against bleeding risk, and having considerable experience in managing patients on warfarin.

3.3.4 Monitoring

Upon initiation, it takes about 2–3 days usually to see an increase on the international normalized ratio (INR) and about 5–7 days to see the full effect of warfarin on INR (corresponding approximately to the amount of time it takes for factor IIa to be depleted). A usual starting dose is 5 mg. Smaller doses such as 2 or 3 mg may be given in patients who are elderly or who are expected to have lesser dose requirements (e.g., CKD patients, patients with lighter body weight, presence of drugs that could raise the INR). Due to the delayed effect of warfarin, it may be overlapped with some faster-acting anticoagulants such as heparin, enoxaparin, or DOACs if immediate anticoagulation is needed.

INR is affected mainly by three factors, namely, drugs including natural supplements, patient's medical condition, and diet and lifestyle. These factors need to be considered when dosing a patient and when an explanation for a subtherapeutic or supratherapeutic INR is being sought.

3.3.5 Adverse effects

The most important adverse effect of warfarin is bleeding. Bleeding risk increases when the INR is >4. The risk of bleed is generally <3% annually if INR is kept between 2 and 3 [1]. If bleeding occurs and warfarin has to be reversed, patients should be given IV Vitamin K and Prothrombin Complex Concentrate (PCC). Fresh frozen plasma (FFP) may also be used as an alternative to PCC but it carries some disadvantages such as delayed administration due to thawing, and infusion of large volumes of fluid [9, 10].

Other notable adverse effects of warfarin include skin necrosis, which occurs 3–8 days after initiation of warfarin [5]. Skin lesions appear due to thrombi in the capillaries and veins. They are usually found in areas rich with fatty tissue such as the breast, abdomen, and extremities. Skin lesion may occur in two types of patients. First is in patients treated with warfarin who have active HIT. Second is in patients who have protein S and/or C deficiency. The exact pathophysiology is not known but may be due to the abrupt drop in protein S and/or C before factors IIa, VIIa, IXa, and Xa drops sufficiently that cause the scale to tip over to the prothrombotic side. In such events, warfarin may be started slowly with concurrent heparin. Stop heparin when INR has reached the therapeutic range [10, 11].

Another adverse effect is purple toe syndrome that occurs 3–10 weeks after initiation of warfarin. The exact pathophysiology is not known but may be due to cholesterol deposits embolizing from the arterioles when the patient develops microbleeds in the atherosclerotic arterioles. The cholesterol emboli could occlude the arteries downstream. It can be reversed when it is discovered early and when warfarin is discontinued. Otherwise, it may lead to gangrene necessitating amputation [5, 11–13].

Other less serious adverse effects include osteoporosis, alopecia, etc. [5, 10]. Warfarin has also been associated with acute kidney injury termed warfarin-related nephropathy.

3.4 Dabigatran

3.4.1 Mechanism of action

Dabigatran is a competitive direct thrombin (factor IIa) inhibitor. It binds to both free and clot-bound thrombin [1, 5, 10, 14]. This is in contrast to heparin which can only bind to free thrombin. As a result, fibrinogen cannot be converted to fibrin. Parenteral direct factor IIa inhibitors have been available in the market before the introduction of dabigatran. Some examples are argatroban, bivalirudin, etc.

3.4.2 ADME

Dabigatran has low oral bioavailability of only 3–7% and is a substrate of P-glycoprotein (P-gp). It comes as a prodrug called dabigatran etexilate that gets hydrolyzed to dabigatran. It reaches its peak concentration about 2 hours after ingestion. Dabigatran is 35% bound to protein and is highly (80%) renally excreted. Dabigatran is 50–60% dialyzable, an important point to take note of especially in cases of toxicity. It has a half-life of 12–17 hours and is dosed twice a day [15, 16] (see **Table 1**).

3.4.3 Clinical use

Dabigatran was the first medication under the new class of medications called novel oral anticoagulants (NOAC) or Direct-acting Oral Anticoagulant (DOAC). Dabigatran is approved for stroke and systemic embolism (SSE) prevention for patients with non-valvular atrial fibrillation, treatment of VTE, and VTE prophylaxis post-hip replacement.

Dabigatran is available in three doses: 75, 110, and 150 mg. Some countries, in the United States, for example, only have 75 and 150 mg. As with the other NOACs, dabigatran can be given without the need for any monitoring of anticoagulation intensity. However, renal function must be monitored carefully as dabigatran is highly renally cleared (80% of the drug).

In terms of efficacy as compared to warfarin for SSE prevention, dabigatran 110 mg has similar efficacy to warfarin titrated to an INR of 2–3. Dabigatran

	Warfarin	Dabigatran	Rivaroxaban	Apixaban	Edoxaban
Target(s)	IIa, VIIa, IXa, Xa	IIa	Xa	Xa	Xa
Prodrug	No	Yes	No	No	No
Bioavailability (%)	80–100	6.5 (pH dependent)	80	50	62
Volume of distribution (L)	10	50–70	50	23	>300
Peak effect	4–5 days	1.5–3 h	2–4 h	1–3 h	1–2 h
Half-life[a]	40 h	12–17 h	5–9 h	9–14 h	10–14 h
Renal elimination	None	80 %	33 %	25 %	35–50 %
Protein binding (%)	>99	35	90	87	55
Dialyzable	No	Yes	No	No	Possible
Interactions	Many	P-gp	3A4, P-gp	3A4, P-gp	P-gp
Coagulation monitoring	Yes	No	No	No	No
Antidote	Vitamin K	Idarucizumab	No	No	No
Lab measure	INR	aPTT TT, ECT	PT Anti-Xa	Anti-Xa	Anti-Xa

[a] Normal renal function

P-gp P glycoprotein, *3A4* cytochrome P450 3A4, *INR* international normalized ratio, *PT* prothrombin time, *aPTT* activated partial thromboplastin time, *TT* thrombin time, *dTT* dilute thrombin time, *ECT* ecarin clotting time

Table 1.
Pharmacokinetic and pharmacodynamic properties of the different oral anticoagulants. Reprint with permission from [16].

150 mg, on the other hand, is superior to warfarin titrated to an INR of 2–3. The superiority is mainly driven by a decrease in stroke events among patients taking dabigatran 150 mg. This is based on the RE-LY (Dabigatran versus Warfarin in Patients with Atrial Fibrillation) trial that led to the approval of dabigatran. In terms of bleeding risk, dabigatran 110 mg has lower overall major bleeding risk, similar gastrointestinal (GI) bleeding risk, and lower intracranial hemorrhage (ICH) compared to warfarin. With regards to dabigatran 150 mg vs. warfarin, dabigatran 150 mg has a similar overall bleeding risk, higher rates of GI bleed, and similar ICH risk compared to warfarin. These have to be taken into consideration when choosing which DOAC is more suitable for a patient [17] (see **Table 2**).

In terms of VTE treatment, dabigatran is not inferior to warfarin in terms of efficacy and safety based on the RE-COVER and RE-COVER II studies [17] (see **Table 3**). One caveat in its use for VTE treatment is that it requires a parenteral lead-in of at least 5 days with UFH or LMWH based on how it was carried out in the studies [19].

3.4.4 Monitoring

No pharmacodynamic monitoring is needed for any of the DOACs including dabigatran. Dabigatran has little effect on prothrombin time (PT) and INR. With regards to the activated partial thromboplastin time (aPTT), a normal aPTT does not exclude the presence of dabigatran. More sensitive tests for dabigatran are Thrombin Time (TT), Ecarin Clotting Time (ECT) and Diluted Thrombin Time (dTT) [20, 21] (see **Table 1**).

3.4.5 Adverse effects

Dabigatran, being a blood thinner, has bleeding as its main side effect. Careful consideration of the bleeding risk factors of the patients needs to be done prior to prescribing dabigatran 150 mg twice daily. History of prior GI bleeding, peptic ulcer disease, colonic angiodysplasia, and other pathologies that predispose a patient to GI bleeding are some practical issues that the prescriber needs to be mindful of. Dyspepsia, abdominal pain, and abdominal discomfort are other side effects that occurred more frequently compared to warfarin [5, 16]. The RE-LY trial has raised concerns about increased myocardial infarction (MI) risk among patients taking dabigatran but the US Food and Drug Administration (FDA) has not found an increase MI risk among patients taking dabigatran in its observational study [22]. Because dabigatran is highly renally cleared, the serum creatinine and creatinine clearance has to be regularly monitored.

3.5 Rivaroxaban

3.5.1 Mechanism of action

Rivaroxaban is the first direct factor Xa inhibitor [16]. It therefore prevents the formation of factor II to factor IIa. It acts one step higher on the coagulation cascade compared to dabigatran. Rivaroxaban is able to bind to both free and clot-bound factor Xa due to its small size (436 g/mol) [10].

3.5.2 ADME

Rivaroxaban has good bioavailability of 66% when taken without food. The bioavailability dramatically increases when it is taken with food to 80–100%.

Characteristics	RE-LY (dabigatran)	ROCKET AF (rivaroxaban)	ARISTOTLE (apixaban)	ENGAGE AF (edoxaban)
Design	Randomized, open label[a]	Randomized, DB/DD	Randomized, DB/DD	Randomized, DB/DD
Dosing	150 mg, 110 mg twice daily	20 mg daily	5 mg twice daily	60 mg, 30 mg daily
Dose adjustment/criteria	No	If CrCl 30–49 mL/min then 15 mg	If ≥2 factors: age ≥80 years, body weight <60 kg, creat ≥1.5 mg/dL then 2.5 mg	If CrCl 30–50 mL/min or weight ≤60 kg or potent P-gp inhibitor[b] then 50 % dose
CrCl exclusion	30 mL/min	30 mL/min	25 mL/min	30 mL/min
$CHADS_2$ score inclusion criteria	≥1	≥2	≥1	≥2
Primary efficacy endpoint	Stroke/TIA and SE	Stroke/TIA and SE	Stroke/TIA and SE	Stroke/TIA and SE
Primary safety endpoint	Major bleeding	Major plus CRNM bleeding	Major bleeding	Major bleeding
Trial size	18,113	14,264	18,201	21,105
Age (years), median (IQR)	72±9[c]	73 (65–78)	70 (63–76)	72 (64–78)
$CHADS_2$ (mean)	2.1	3.5	2.1	2.8
$CHADS_2$ ≥3 (%)	32	87	30	53
Heart failure	32	62	35	57
Stroke/TIA or SE	20[d]	55	19	28
Median follow-up (years)	2.0	1.9	1.8	2.8
Early discontinuation				
DOAC (%)	20.7/21.2	35.4	25.3	33.0/34.3
VKA (%)	16.6	34.6	27.5	34.4

CRNM clinically relevant non-major bleeding, *DB/DD* double blind, double dummy, *IQR* interquartile range, *DOAC* direct oral anticoagulant, *SE* systemic embolism, *TIA* transient ischemic attack, *VKA* vitamin K antagonist, *CrCl* creatinine clearance

[a] Patients were unblended with respect to dabigatran or warfarin assignment; however, all investigators, coordinating center members, the steering committee, the event adjudication committee, and the sponsor were blinded during event ascertainment and analyses

[b] Strong P-gp inhibitors such as dronedarone, quinidine, or verapamil

[c] Mean±SD

[d] No data on SE

DOAC vs VKA HR (95 % CI)	RE-LY[a] (dabigatran) 110 mg 150 mg	ROCKET AF (rivaroxaban) 20 mg	ARISTOTLE (apixaban) 5 mg	ENGAGE AF-TIMI 48 (edoxaban) 30 mg 60 mg
Ischemic stroke	1.11 (0.89–1.40)[a]	0.94 (0.75–1.17)	0.92 (0.74–1.13)	***1.41 (1.19–1.67) p < 0.001***
	0.76 (0.60–0.98)[a] p = 0.03			1.00 (0.83–1.19)
Systemic embolism	Not reported	**0.23 (0.09–0.61) p = 0.003**	0.87 (0.44–1.75)	1.24 (0.72–2.15)
				0.65 (0.34–1.24)
Hemorrhagic stroke	**0.31 (0.17–0.56) p < .0001**	**0.59 (0.37–0.93 p = 0.024)**	**0.51 (0.35–0.75) p < 0.001**	**0.33 (0.22–0.50) p < 0.001**
	0.26 (0.14–0.49 p < 0.001			**0.54 (0.38–0.77) p < 0.001**
Major bleed	**0.80 (0.69–0.93) p = 0.003**	1.04 (0.90–1.20)	**0.69 (0.60–0.80) p < 0.001**	**0.47 (0.41–0.55) p < 0.001**
	0.93 (0.81–1.07) p = 0.3			**0.80 (0.71–0.91) p < 0.001**
Intracranial bleed	**0.31 (0.20–0.47) p < 0.001**	**0.67 (0.47–0.93) p = 0.02**	**0.42 (0.30–0.58) p < 0.001**	**0.30 (0.21–0.43) p < 0.001**
	0.40 (0.27–0.60) p < 0.001			**0.47 (0.34–0.63) p < 0.001**
Gastrointestinal bleed	1.10 (0.86–1.41)	***3.2 vs 2.2[b] p < 0.001***	0.89 (0.70–1.15)	**0.67 (0.53–0.83) p < 0.001**
	1.50 (1.19–1.89) p < 0.001			***1.23 (1.02–1.50) p = 0.03***
All-cause mortality	0.91 (0.80–1.03)	0.85 (0.70–1.02)	**0.89 (0.80–0.98) p = 0.047**	**0.87 (0.79–0.96) p = 0.006**
	0.88 (0.77–1.00) p = 0.051			0.92 (0.83–1.01)
Cardiovascular mortality	0.90 (0.77–1.06)[a]	0.89 (0.73–1.10)	0.89 (0.76–1.04)	**0.85 (0.76–0.96) p = 0.008**
	0.85 (0.72–0.99)[a] p = 0.04			**0.86 (0.77–0.97) p = 0.013**

Bold font indicates significantly better result of DOAC in relation to warfarin. Bold and italic font indicates significantly worse result of DOAC compared to warfarin

[a] RE-LY reported relative risk instead of hazard ratio (HR); ischemic or uncertain stroke instead ischemic stroke, and vascular mortality instead cardiovascular mortality

[b] Incidence/year (%), HR not reported

Table 2.
Characteristics, efficacy, and safety data of warfarin vs. DOACs for stroke and systemic embolism prevention in patients with non-valvular atrial fibrillation. Adapted from [31] under Creative Commons (CC BY) Attribution 4.0 International License.

Rivaroxaban reaches its peak concentration about 2–4 hours after ingestion. Rivaroxaban is highly protein bound at 95%. Two-thirds of the drug is degraded by the liver via CYP3A4 and CYP3A5, and CYP2J2 to a lesser extent, half of which is then excreted renally and the other half is excreted by the hepato-biliary route into the feces. The remaining one-third of the drug is excreted renally. Rivaroxaban is a P-gp substrate both at the gut and at the kidney, hence

Trial	Dabigatran		Rivaroxaban		Apixaban	Edoxaban
	RE-COVER	RE-COVER II	EINSTEIN-DVT	EINSTEIN-PE	AMPLIFY	Hokusai-VTE
Year	2009	2014	2010	2012	2013	2013
Design	Double-blind	Double-blind	Open-label	Open-label	Double-blind	Double-blind
# of patients	2539	2589	3449	4832	5395	8292
LMHW/heparin bridge	Yes	Yes	No	No	No	Yes
Treatment protocol	Dabigatran 150 mg BID	Dabigatran 150 mg BID	Rivaroxaban 15 mg BID for 3 weeks; then 20 mg daily	Rivaroxaban 15 mg BID for 3 weeks; then 20 mg daily	Apixaban 10 mg BID for 7 days; then 5 mg BID	Edoxaban 60mg daily; or 30 mg daily for patients w/CrCl 30–50 ml/min, weight ≤ 60 kg, or receiving P-glycoprotein inhibitors
Duration of therapy (months)	6	6	3, 6, or 12	3, 6, or 12	6	≤ 12
Primary efficacy outcome	Recurrent VTE and related death	Recurrent VTE and related death	Recurrent VTE	Recurrent VTE	Recurrent VTE and related death	Recurrent VTE and related death
Event rate of primary efficacy outcome: NOAC vs. VKA	2.4% vs. 2.1%	2.3% vs. 2.2%	2.1% vs. 3.0%	2.1% vs. 1.8%	2.3% vs. 2.7%	3.2% vs. 3.5%
Hazard ratio (HR), 95% confidence interval (CI)	1.10 (0.65–1.84) $P<0.001$	1.08 (0.64–1.80) $P<0.001$	0.68 (0.44–1.04) $P<0.001$	1.12 (0.75–1.68) $P = 0.003$	0.84 (0.60–1.18) $P<0.001$	0.89 (0.70–1.13) $P<0.001$
Primary safety outcome	Major bleed	Major bleed	Major or CRNM bleed	Major or CRNM bleed	Major bleed	Major or CRNM bleed
Event rate of primary safety outcome: NOAC vs. VKA	1.6% vs. 1.9%	1.2% vs. 1.7%	8.1% vs. 8.1%	10.3% vs. 11.4%	0.6% vs. 1.8%	8.5% vs. 10.3%
HR, 95% CI	0.82 (0.45–1.48)	0.69 (0.36–1.32)	0.97 (0.76–1.22) $P = 0.77$	0.90 (0.76–1.07) $P = 0.23$	0.31 (0.17–0.55) $P<0.001$	0.81 (0.71–0.94) $P = 0.004$

BID twice daily dosing, *CrCl* creatinine clearance, *CRNM* clinically relevant nonmajor, *DVT* deep vein thrombosis, *LMWH* low molecular weight heparin, *NOAC* non vitamin K oral anticoagulant, *PE* pulmonary embolism, *VKA* vitamin K antagonist, *VTE* venous thromboembolism

Table 3.
Efficacy and safety data of DOACs venous thromboembolism treatment. Adapted from [18] under Creative Commons (CC BY) Attribution 4.0 International License.

drug–drug interaction between rivaroxaban and P-gp substrates, inhibitors, or inducers must be taken note of. The half-life of rivaroxaban is about 5–9 hours for the younger patients. It has a longer half-life of 11–13 hours among the elderly [15, 16] (see **Table 1**).

3.5.3 Clinical use

Rivaroxaban comes in various strengths of 2.5, 10, 15, and 20 mg tablets. It is approved for stroke and systemic embolism prevention in patients with non-valvular AF, VTE treatment and prophylaxis including patients who had Total Knee Replacement (TKR) and Total Hip Replacement (THR), and for cardiovascular risk reduction among patients with Coronary Artery Disease (CAD) or Peripheral Artery Disease (PAD) in the United States.

For SSE prevention in patients with non-valvular AF, rivaroxaban has demonstrated non-inferiority both in efficacy and safety compared to warfarin. Careful examination of the data from the Rivaroxaban versus Warfarin in Nonvalvular Atrial Fibrillation (ROCKET AF) trial shows that rivaroxaban has higher GI bleeding rates but lower ICH rates compared to warfarin [23] (see **Table 2**).

For VTE treatment, rivaroxaban is non-inferior as well compared to warfarin (see **Table 3**). However, the initial treatment dose is 15 mg twice daily × 3 weeks followed by 20 mg daily [18]. The reason for the twice daily dosing is likely due to the need for a higher concentration for clot resolution and prevention of further propagation, knowing that the risk of VTE occurrence is highest during the first 3–4 weeks [24].

At a dose of 2.5 mg twice daily in combination with aspirin and either clopidogrel or ticlopidine, rivaroxaban has shown small 16% relative risk reduction, or 1.6% absolute risk reduction (NNT = 63) for death due to cardiovascular causes, MI, or stroke. This is at the backdrop of higher bleeding events (NNH = 83 for TIMI major bleeding events not associated with CABG) [25]. Patients subjected to rivaroxaban 2.5 mg twice daily need to be carefully selected.

3.5.4 Monitoring

No routine laboratory monitoring is needed for rivaroxaban for its pharmacodynamic effect. Rivaroxaban may affect PT/INR depending on the reagent used; elevated PT/INR may signal the presence of the drug but rivaroxaban cannot be excluded even if the PT/INR is normal [15, 20, 21]. Rivaroxaban may affect aPTT but less so compared to PT/INR. The best test to measure for the effect of the drug is via anti-factor Xa assay [20, 21], which is not routinely available in most hospital laboratories. Patient's serum creatinine and creatinine clearance should be periodically monitored to see if dose adjustment might be needed.

3.5.5 Adverse effects

Bleeding is the adverse effect of utmost concern among patients started on rivaroxaban. Patients with history of GI bleeding should select other oral anticoagulants besides rivaroxaban due to its higher GI bleed risk when studied against warfarin.

3.6 Apixaban

3.6.1 Mechanism of action

Similar to rivaroxaban, apixaban is also a direct factor Xa inhibitor [16, 26]. It thus inhibits one step higher on the coagulation cascade compared to dabigatran. It binds to both free and clot-bound factor Xa.

3.6.2 ADME

Apixaban has a bioavailability of 50% and is an active drug itself. It is also a substrate of P-gp. It reaches peak concentration 2–4 hours after ingestion. It is highly protein bound as well at 87%. Apixaban is cleared both via renal and non-renal pathway. Fifty percent of the drug is excreted into the feces unchanged, 27% is also excreted in the urine unchanged. The remaining (~25%) undergoes metabolism by CYP3A4 and by other minor CYP enzymes such as CYP1A2, 2J2, 2C8, 2C9, and 2C19. It has a half-life of 9–14 hours [15, 16, 19, 26] (see **Table 1**).

3.6.3 Clinical use

Apixaban is approved in the US for SSE in patients with non-valvular AF, VTE treatment and prophylaxis, including patients' post-TKR and post-THR, and for long-term recurrent VTE prophylaxis. It comes in two strengths of 2.5 and 5 mg tablets.

In the Apixaban versus Warfarin in Patients with Atrial Fibrillation (ARISTOTLE) trial, apixaban demonstrated superiority over warfarin titrated to an INR of 2–3 with relative risk reduction of 21%, absolute risk reduction of 0.33% giving an NNT of 303. This statistically significant result is driven mainly by a decrease in hemorrhagic stroke rates. In terms of bleeding events, apixaban demonstrated 31% less bleeding compared to warfarin, mainly driven by decrease in ICH and bleeding other than GI bleeding rates. Of note, apixaban has similar GI bleeding rates versus warfarin. Apixaban is used at a dose of 5 mg twice daily for SSE prevention (see **Table 2**). The dose is reduced to 2.5 mg twice daily if two out of the three following criteria are met: weight of ≤60 kg, serum creatinine of >1.5 mg/dl, or age of ≥80 years old according to the drug label. It should be noted that patients with CrCl of <25 ml/min are not included in the trial and hence other countries do not allow use of apixaban in patients with CrCl of <25 ml/min [27]. However, in the US, apixaban can be used at a dose of 2.5 mg twice daily even in patients with end-stage renal disease, including patients on dialysis, based on pharmacokinetic modeling.

For the treatment of VTE, apixaban is non-inferior to warfarin but has lower bleeding episodes (see **Table 3**). Apixaban is started at a dose of 10 mg twice daily for 7 days followed by 5 mg twice daily [19, 26]. Similarly, apixaban should be avoided in patients with CrCl of <25 ml/min as these patients were excluded in the trial.

3.6.4 Monitoring

Apixaban does not require any laboratory monitoring as well. PT/INR is even less sensitive to apixaban compared to rivaroxaban. Anti-factor Xa assay specifically calibrated to apixaban is a sensitive test that could detect the presence and could give the quantity of the drug present in the sample. However, anti-factor Xa assay for DOACs are not readily available in most hospital laboratories [20, 21, 26].

3.6.5 Adverse effects

Patients on apixaban need to watch for bleeding, though apixaban has a better safety profile than warfarin.

3.7 Edoxaban

3.7.1 Mechanism of action

Edoxaban is also a direct factor Xa inhibitor, like rivaroxaban and apixaban [16].

3.7.2 ADME

Edoxaban is 62% bioavailable and is a P-gp substrate as well. Peak concentration occurs 1–2 hours after ingestion of edoxaban. Edoxaban is cleared both renally and non-renally in a 50-50 manner. Fifty percent of the drug is metabolized hepatically via hydrolysis. Only 4% of the drug is metabolized by CYP3A4. The remaining 50% of the drug is excreted renally. It has a half-life of 10–14 hours [15, 19, 28] (see **Table 1**).

3.7.3 Clinical use

Edoxaban is approved both for SSE prevention in patients with non-valvular AF and VTE treatment. In the Edoxaban versus Warfarin in Patients with Atrial Fibrillation (ENGAGE AF-TIMI 48) trial, edoxaban has shown to be non-inferior to warfarin for SSE prevention [28] (see **Table 2**). However, a separate analysis that was published shows that at CrCl of >95 ml/min, edoxaban is not as protective as warfarin against SSE. Patients with CrCl >95 ml/min have lower edoxaban concentration likely due to higher clearance of the drug among those with CrCl of 95 ml/min [29]. Hence, edoxaban is not approved by the US FDA for use among patients with CrCl of >95 ml/min. In terms of bleeding episodes, edoxaban has lesser bleeding risk than warfarin. Edoxaban comes in 30 and 60 mg doses. The 30 mg dose is used if patients have CrCL of 30–50 ml/min, weighs ≤60 kg, or is on verapamil, quinidine, or dronedarone (medication that are strong P-gp inhibitors) [28].

For the treatment of VTE, edoxaban is non-inferior to warfarin in terms of efficacy and has a lesser bleeding occurrence (see **Table 3**). There is no FDA recommendation whether it should be avoided in patients with CrCl > 95 ml/min due to lack of studies. However, it would seem prudent to also do the same for patients with VTE [18].

3.7.4 Monitoring

Edoxaban does not require monitoring like other DOACs. Similar to rivaroxaban and apixaban, PT/INR has low sensitivity towards edoxaban's pharmacodynamic effect and is therefore not a good laboratory test to check on the presence of the drug. Anti-factor Xa assay calibrated to edoxaban remains to be the most sensitive test for edoxaban so far [20, 21, 28].

3.7.5 Adverse effects

Edoxaban has demonstrated lesser bleeding risk compared to warfarin in the clinical phase III studies.

4. Conclusion

The use of anticoagulants requires holistic evaluation of the patient and careful balancing of the thrombotic and bleeding risks of the patient. Understanding the pharmacology, pharmacodynamics, pharmacokinetics, and clinical evidence behind the use of these drugs will help the clinician in selecting the best therapy for the patient.

Conflict of interest

The author has no conflict of interest to declare.

Notes/thanks/other declarations

None.

Author details

Hobart Owen Ng Tsai
Khoo Teck Puat Hospital, Singapore

*Address all correspondence to: hngtsai@gmail.com

References

[1] Hilal-Dandan R, Brunton LL. Goodman and Gilman's Manual of Pharmacology and Therapeutics. 2nd ed. China: McGraw Hill Professional; 2014. pp. 523-543

[2] Adams RL, Bird RJ. Review article: Coagulation cascade and therapeutics update: Relevance to nephrology. Part 1: Overview of coagulation, thrombophilias and history of anticoagulants. Nephrology (Carlton, Vic.). 2009;**14**(5):462-470. DOI: 10.1111/j.1440-1797.2009.01128.x

[3] Garcia DA, Baglin TP, Weitz JI, Samama MM. Parenteral anticoagulants: Antithrombotic therapy and prevention of thrombosis, 9th ed: American College of Chest Physicians Evidence-Based Clinical Practice Guidelines. Chest. 2012;**141**(2 Suppl):e24S-e43S. DOI: 10.1378/chest.11-2291

[4] Smythe MA, Priziola J, Dobesh PP, Wirth D, Cuker A, Wittkowsky AK. Guidance for the practical management of the heparin anticoagulants in the treatment of venous thromboembolism. Journal of Thrombosis and Thrombolysis. 2016;**41**(1):165-186. DOI: 10.1007/s11239-015-1315-2

[5] Maddali S, Biring T, Bluhm J, Kopecky S, Krueger K, Larson T, et al. Institute for Clinical Systems Improvement. Antithrombotic Therapy Supplement. Updated February 2013

[6] DiPiro JT, Talbert RL, Yee GC, et al. Pharmacotherapy. A Pathophysiologic Approach. USA: McGraw Hill Professional; 2008. pp. 331-371

[7] Cuker A, Arepally GM, Chong BH, et al. American Society of Hematology 2018 guidelines for management of venous thromboembolism: heparin-induced thrombocytopenia. Blood Advances. 2018;**2**(22):3360-3392

[8] Witt DM, Nieuwlaat R, Clark NP, et al. American Society of Hematology 2018 guidelines for management of venous thromboembolism: optimal management of anticoagulation therapy. Blood Advances. 2018;**2**(22):3257-3291. DOI: 10.1182/bloodadvances.2018024893

[9] Murphy JE. Clinical pharmacokinetics. American Society of Health-System; 2012

[10] Ageno W, Gallus AS, Wittkowsky A, Crowther M, Hylek EM, Palareti G. Oral anticoagulant therapy: Antithrombotic therapy and prevention of thrombosis, 9th ed: American College of Chest Physicians Evidence-Based Clinical Practice Guidelines. Chest. 2012;**141**(Suppl. 2):e44S-e88S. DOI: 10.1378/chest.11-2292

[11] Hirsh J, Fuster V, Ansell J, Halperin JL. American Heart Association/American College of Cardiology Foundation guide to warfarin therapy. Circulation. 2003;**107**(12):1692-1711. DOI: 10.1161/01.CIR.0000063575.17904.4E

[12] Devalia K, Darby C. Purple toe syndrome. European Journal of Vascular and Endovascular Surgery. 2006;**31**:99-100. DOI: 10.1016/j.ejvs.2005.04.008

[13] Cakebread HE, Knight HM, Gajendragadkar PR, Cooper JP. Warfarin-induced purple toe syndrome successfully treated with apixaban. BML Case Reports. 2014;**2014**:1-2. DOI: 10.1136/bcr-2014-205320

[14] Ganetsky M, Babu KM, Salhanick SD, Brown RS, Boyer EW. Dabigatran: review of pharmacology and management of bleeding complications of this novel oral anticoagulant. Journal of Medical Toxicology. 2011;7(4):281-287. DOI: 10.1007/s13181-011-0178-y

[15] Steffel J, Verhamme P, Potpara TS, et al. The 2018 European Heart Rhythm Association Practical Guide on the use of non-vitamin K antagonist oral anticoagulants in patients with atrial fibrillation. European Heart Journal. 2018;**39**(16):1330-1393. DOI: 10.1093/eurheartj/ehy136

[16] Nutescu EA, Burnett A, Fanikos J, Spinler S, Wittkowsky A. Erratum to: Pharmacology of anticoagulants used in the treatment of venous thromboembolism. Journal of Thrombosis and Thrombolysis. 2016;**42**(2):296-311. DOI: 10.1007/s11239-016-1363-2

[17] Connolly SJ, Ezekowitz MD, Yusuf S, et al. Dabigatran versus warfarin in patients with atrial fibrillation. The New England Journal of Medicine. 2009;**361**(12):1139-1151. DOI: 10.1056/NEJMoa0905561

[18] Bromley A, Plitt A. A review of the role of non-vitamin K oral anticoagulants in the acute and long-term treatment of venous thromboembolism. Cardiology and Therapy. 2018;**7**(1):1-13. DOI: 10.1007/s40119-018-0107-0

[19] Burnett AE, Mahan CE, Vazquez SR, Oertel LB, Garcia DA, Ansell J. Guidance for the practical management of the direct oral anticoagulants (DOACs) in VTE treatment. Journal of Thrombosis and Thrombolysis. 2016;**41**(1):206-232. DOI: 10.1007/s11239-015-1310-7

[20] Douxfils J, Ageno W, Samama CM, et al. Laboratory testing in patients treated with direct oral anticoagulants: A practical guide for clinicians. Journal of Thrombosis and Haemostasis. 2018;**16**(2):209-219. DOI: 10.1111/jth.13912

[21] Conway SE, Hwang AY, Ponte CD, Gums JG. Laboratory and clinical monitoring of direct acting oral anticoagulants: What clinicians need to know. Pharmacotherapy. 2017;**37**(2):236-248. DOI: 10.1002/phar.1884

[22] Food and Drug Administration. FDA study of Medicare patients finds risks lower for stroke and death but higher for gastrointestinal bleeding with Pradaxa (dabigatran) compared to warfarin [press release]; 2014

[23] Patel MR, Mahaffey KW, Garg J, et al. Rivaroxaban versus warfarin in nonvalvular atrial fibrillation. The New England Journal of Medicine. 2011;**365**(10):883-891. DOI: 10.1056/NEJMoa1009638

[24] Kubitza D, Berkowitz SD, Misselwitz F. Evidence-based development and rationale for once-daily rivaroxaban dosing regimens across multiple indications. Clinical and Applied Thrombosis/Hemostasis. 2016;**22**(5):412-422. DOI: 10.1177/1076029616631427

[25] Mega JL, Braunwald E, Wiviott SD, et al. Rivaroxaban in patients with a recent acute coronary syndrome. The New England Journal of Medicine. 2012;**366**(1):9-19. DOI: 10.1056/NEJMoa1112277

[26] Ward C, Conner G, Donnan G, Gallus A, Mcrae S. Practical management of patients on apixaban: A consensus guide. Thrombosis Journal. 2013;**11**(1):27. DOI: 10.1186/1477-9560-11-27

[27] Granger CB, Alexander JH, Mcmurray JJ, et al. Apixaban versus warfarin in patients with atrial fibrillation. The New England Journal of Medicine. 2011;**365**(11):981-992. DOI: 10.1056/NEJMoa1107039

[28] Stacy ZA, Call WB, Hartmann AP, Peters GL, Richter SK. Edoxaban: A comprehensive review of the pharmacology and clinical data for the

management of atrial fibrillation and venous thromboembolism. Cardiology and Therapy. 2016;**5**(1):1-18. DOI: 10.1007/s40119-016-0058-2

[29] Bohula EA, Giugliano RP, Ruff CT, et al. Impact of renal function on outcomes with edoxaban in the ENGAGE AF-TIMI 48 trial. Circulation. 2016;**134**(1):24-36. DOI: 10.1161/CIRCULATIONAHA.116.022361

[30] Davie EW. A brief historical review of the waterfall/cascade of blood coagulation. The Journal of Biological Chemistry. 2003;**278**(51):50819-50832. DOI: 10.1074/jbc.X300009200

[31] Schaefer JK, Mcbane RD, Wysokinski WE. How to choose appropriate direct oral anticoagulant for patient with nonvalvular atrial fibrillation. Annals of Hematology. 2016;**95**(3):437-449

Chapter 3

Update on Mechanisms, Pathogenicity, Heterogeneity of Presentation, and Laboratory Diagnosis of Heparin-Induced Thrombocytopenia

Jean Amiral and Anne Marie Vissac

Abstract

Heparin-induced thrombocytopenia (HIT) is the most life-threatening adverse effect of heparin therapy and is provoked by the development of drug-dependent antibodies. It occurs more frequently in patients with cardiac or orthopedic surgery or severe circulatory diseases, and the risk depends on the patient pathological status. As heparin is an anticoagulant used for treating thrombotic events or their risk, this iatrogenic complication has a paradoxal effect as it can induce thromboembolic diseases, frequently associated to severe morbidity or fatal outcomes. Diagnosis involves clinical evaluation of disease probability and laboratory tools for testing the presence of heparin-dependent antibodies with immunoassays or their capability to activate platelets with functional assays. Antibodies developed when stoichiometric complexes of platelet factor 4 (PF4) with heparin are formed during therapy. In few cases non-platelet factor 4 antigens can be involved. Antibodies can remain asymptomatic, but pathogenicity occurs in the presence of high concentrations of IgG isotype antibodies, with high avidity: they target and activate platelets or endothelial cells exposing heparin-PF4 (HPF4) complexes and produce thrombocytopenia and sometimes thrombosis. Risk factors which favor the development of antibodies and their pathological effect are discussed. The present understanding of mechanisms underlying disease development and diagnostic strategies of this heparin adverse effect is presented.

Keywords: platelet factor 4, heparin, antibodies, pathogenicity, thrombosis, thrombocytopenia, diagnosis

1. Introduction

The major adverse effect of heparin therapy concerns probably the development of thrombocytopenia and thromboembolic complications, which are directly caused by the drug itself [1–6]. This heparin paradox is associated with a characteristic platelet fall and thrombosis in some heparin-treated patients, especially when unfractionated heparin (UFH) is used, but it can also occur with low molecular weight heparin (LMWH) therapy. The patient's clinical context can favor the development of this iatrogenic complication, called heparin-induced thrombocytopenia (HIT) without or with associated thrombosis (HITT). When this complication occurs, it requires an immediate management with the withdrawal of heparin and use of an alternative anticoagulant [7–11]. If incorrectly managed, it can rapidly cause severe burden and become life-threatening. This complication is reported to occur in about 1–5% of patients treated with UFH and 0.2–0.5% of those treated with LMWH, but the incidence highly depends on the clinical context [1, 3, 5, 6]. Cardiology or orthopedic surgery, trauma, circulatory diseases, and the presence of tumors are increased risk factors for that disease. A recent meta-analysis in the USA reported a different HIT/HITT incidence and clinical association than that usually accepted but shows that it remains a critical clinical issue in hospitals [5]. The first alert signal for HIT is a platelet count drop by more than 30–50% between two successive measures, occurring between 5 and 15 days following the onset of heparin therapy, in the absence of any other thrombocytopenia cause (**Table 1**). However, platelet fall can develop earlier if patients have been exposed to heparin during the 3 months preceding the treatment. The mechanisms producing HIT involve the generation of a heparin-dependent antibody, usually of the IgG isotype (but IgA and IgM isotypes can also be present). This antibody has been demonstrated to be targeted to complexes of heparin and platelet factor 4 (PF4) in most of the cases [12, 13], but non-PF4 antigens can be present in some atypical patients [14–17]. Frequently, heparin-dependent antibodies, including IgG isotypes, are asymptomatic [18, 19]. They are symptomatic and harmful only in a few subsets of affected patients. What renders the antibodies pathogenic in those patients is not totally understood, but some evidence becomes available. IgG isotypes present at high concentration, and with high avidity, provoke frequently the development of disease [19, 20]. Clinical diagnosis and laboratory diagnosis are of high importance to rapidly identify the patients with an active disease and treat them [6, 8, 21–24]. It includes a multiple strategy approach:

1. early detection of patients with thrombocytopenia

2. evaluation of their HIT clinical score

3. testing for the presence of heparin-dependent antibodies with immunoassays

4. checking the capability of these antibodies to activate platelets in a heparin-dependent mode [25].

It is of essence to duly characterize patients with HIT: if this complication is excluded, it is not necessary to deprive them from heparin, as it is the most effective anticoagulant in many acute conditions. Conversely, if HIT/HITT is confirmed, it is

• Clinical context with blood activation
• Cardiac/orthopedic surgery
• Malignancy
• Autoimmune disorders
• UFH > LMWH
• Heparin therapy duration (≥5 days)
• Re-exposure to heparin <100 days

Table 1.
Risk factors for HIT development during heparin therapy.

mandatory to not reintroduce any heparin treatment and to switch to an alternative anticoagulation. In this book chapter, we will present and discuss the following: (a) the present understandings of conditions which can favor development of heparin-dependent antibodies in heparin-treated patients; (b) why antibodies generate HIT or HITT only in a few subset of patients; (c) the mechanisms of action of these antibodies, as they are presently understood; (d) the available laboratory tools and their indications; (e) the diagnostic strategy for rapidly characterizing patients at risk; (f) the occurrence of atypical presentations of HIT in patients with pre-existing antibodies to PF4 or to interleukin 8 (IL8) or with antibodies to protamine sulfate (PrS); and (g) cross-reactivity of the various polysaccharide anticoagulants in immunoassays and functional methods. This chapter mainly focuses on antibodies generated to heparin-PF4 (HPF4) complexes, which concern most of the patients with HIT/HITT, but other non-PF4 antigens can be involved in few cases and will be rapidly discussed.

2. Development of heparin-induced thrombocytopenia

Heparin-dependent antibodies develop in many patients treated with UFH or LMWH. Their incidence is higher in patients undergoing extracorporeal circulation (ECC) for cardiopulmonary bypass (CPB) or extracorporeal membrane oxygenation (ECMO) [5, 26, 27]. Antibodies' development is not rare during heparin therapy, but they are often of the IgM isotype with a rapid reversal without any clinical incidence [18, 19]. They can also be of the IgA or IgG isotypes, and the three isotypes are associated in many patients and are frequently asymptomatic. IgGs have been demonstrated to be those which can become pathogenic, especially when present at high concentration, with high affinity for their target heparin-dependent antigen [19, 25]. A subset of the IgG isotype heparin-dependent antibodies can then activate platelets [20], which induce thrombocytopenia, platelet aggregation, and sometimes thrombosis. HIT was first characterized for the white thrombus formed in arteries (platelets and white blood cells), when patients with this complication were first identified, but there is evidence now that arterial (about 30% of cases) or venous (about 70% of cases) thrombosis can occur [28]. Skin necrosis at the injection site or elsewhere, or thrombosis, frequently at limb extremities, is often observed, but thrombosis can occur at many different sites.

In addition to platelet activation, heparin-dependent antibodies can induce activation of endothelial cells (ECs) and of monocytes, and they can release tissue factor (TF) from these cells, which contribute to thrombosis [29–31]. Platelet-leukocyte aggregates are also formed and contribute to thrombogenicity. When this multiple blood activation process is initiated, it is enhanced at pathological sites where platelet and white blood cells can be chemo-attracted and accumulate with a high density. If blood activation and prothrombotic process are strong enough to overwhelm the antithrombotic body's defenses, thrombus formation occurs. The first clinical warning for HIT is the occurrence of thrombocytopenia, with a characteristic time kinetics from the onset of therapy, when other causes of decreased platelet counts are excluded [6, 25, 28]. Platelet fall typically occurs between 5 and 15 days following the initiation of treatment, as shown in **Figure 1**, except if patients already received heparin within the 100 preceding days or in the rare cases with pre-existing anti-PF4 antibodies. Thrombocytopenia can then develop earlier and possibly just at the onset of heparin therapy. In HIT/HITT thrombocytopenia is usually moderate, between 20 and 100 giga platelets per liter (G/L), and it is rarely very severe (<10 G/L). When it develops, the clinical probability for HIT/HITT

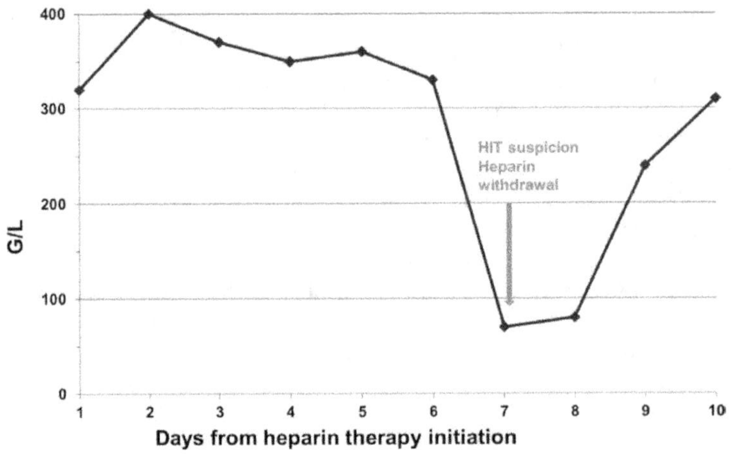

Figure 1.
Typical platelet count kinetics in heparin-treated patients who develop heparin-dependent antibodies responsible for heparin-induced thrombocytopenia.

Quote	Points (0, 1, or 2 for each of 4 categories: maximum possible score = 8)		
Score	2	1	0
Thrombocytopenia	>50% fall from baseline or platelet nadir 20 to 100 x 10⁹/L	30 to 50% fall from baseline or platelet nadir 10 to 19 x 10⁹/L	Fall <30% from baseline or platelet nadir <10x10⁹/L
Timing of platelet count fall or other sequelae	Clear onset between days 5 and 10, or less than 1 day (if heparin exposure within past 100 days).	Consistent with immunization but not clear (e.g., missing platelet counts) or onset of thrombocytopenia after day 10	Platelet count falls too early (without recent heparin exposure)
Thrombosis or other sequelae (e.g., skin lesions)	New thrombosis; skin necrosis; post heparin bolus acute systemic reaction	Progressive or recurrent thrombosis; erythematous skin lesions; suspected thrombosis not yet proven	None
oTher cause for thrombocytopenia	No other cause for platelet count fall is evident	Possible other cause is evident	Definite other cause is evident
Pretest probability score: 6 to 8 = High; 4 to 5 = Intermediate; 0-3 = Low			
Adapted from Warkentin TE. Br J Haematol. 2003;121-535-55.			

Table 2.
The pretest probability for HIT based on the 4Ts score.

must be evaluated. It is an important criterion for estimating the risk to develop this complication in heparin-treated patients, and various pretest methods for estimating disease risk are available. The most frequently used is the 4Ts score [28], which considers four major criteria: the presence of thrombocytopenia, the timing of platelet count fall, the occurrence of new thrombosis or sequelae, and the investigation of other causes of thrombocytopenia. For each criterion, a score from 0 to 2 is given, as shown in **Table 2**. It allows to classify patients from 0 to 8 (risk is low for 0–3, intermediate for 4–5, and high for ≥6, indicating an elevated disease probability). In cardiology patients with ECC, thrombocytopenia is frequently observed, and HIT can be identified when a biphasic platelet count kinetics is present: in the absence of HIT, thrombocytopenia is progressively corrected, but, if present, platelet count starts to increase and falls again when symptomatic antibodies develop [27].

DOI: http://dx.doi.org/10.5772/intechopen.86475

Other HIT clinical evaluation approaches have been proposed (such as the expert score), but the 4Ts score remains the most widely used. When HIT is suspected, heparin treatment must be stopped and replaced by another anticoagulant. The possible drugs which can be used include argatroban, direct oral anticoagulants (DOACs), danaparoid sodium, fondaparinux, and bivalirudin [7, 9–11, 32, 33]. Nevertheless, if HIT is excluded, heparin can be reintroduced, as it can be of full benefit for the patient, especially in cardiac surgery and circulatory diseases. Establishing rapidly a safe and reliable diagnosis of HIT is then of essence for the right management of patients [6, 25, 28].

3. Heparin-dependent antibodies in clinical settings

HIT/HITT occurs in some of the patients who develop heparin-dependent antibodies, a major risk factor for the disease occurrence. In most of the cases, they are targeted to stoichiometric complexes of heparin and PF4 (HPF4) and are of the IgG isotype but are the only ones present in few patients with atypical HIT/HITT antibodies to IL8 or to PrS [12, 14, 15, 17]. In rare cases, the antibody specificity remains non-identified, although patients present the suggestive clinical complication of heparin therapy. What causes the heparin-dependent antibodies' generation is not yet fully understood, but drug immunogenicity tends to develop when heparin forms complexes with its high-affinity binding blood protein, PF4, a chemokine from the CXC family [34–36], and eventually IL8 [37, 38]. In healthy individuals, PF4 is normally present at very low concentrations in blood circulation (<10 ng/ml). It is released from platelets' α-granules upon activation or aggregation, as a complex of eight PF4 tetramers with a platelet proteoglycan dimer, with a molecular weight (MW) of about 350 kDa. This complex is rapidly cleared from circulation as PF4 is captured by endothelial cells' glycosaminoglycans (GAGs) and

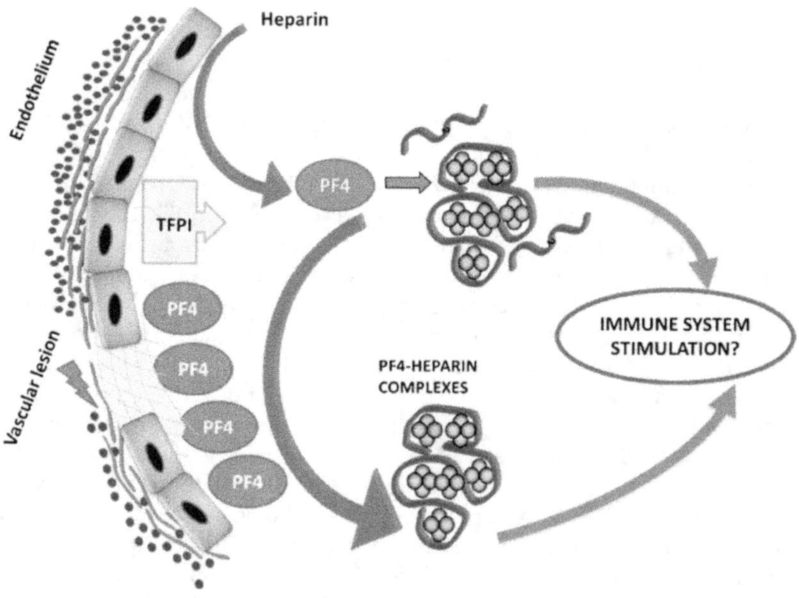

Figure 2.
At the onset of heparin therapy, TFPI and PF4 "storage pool" are displaced from endothelial cells and released into blood circulation. Heparin complexes with PF4, and this can stimulate the immune system (especially if heparin and PF4 stoichiometric concentrations are met), and antibodies to these complexes are generated.

remains in this endothelial storage pool. In patients with inflammation or blood activation, PF4 concentrations can be much higher, either in blood circulation or on the endothelial storage pool. In addition, at pathological sites, platelets and white blood cells can be chemo-attracted and stimulated. Much higher PF4 concentrations can be present at these sites. At the onset of heparin therapy, PF4, which has a higher affinity for this drug than for GAGs or physiological proteoglycans, forms complexes with it, as presented in **Figure 2**. In some circumstances these complexes can activate the immune system and induce the generation of antibodies. The immune response can be innate, mediated via the toll-like receptors, and adaptive with a T cell-mediated response, followed by the generation of antibodies. The three isotypes (IgG, IgA, or IgM) can be present [13, 19], but IgGs are formed very rapidly, which is unusual in the early stage of the immune response, and IgGs can become rapidly pathogenic [19]. In rare cases, only IgA (especially in patients with cancer) or IgM isotypes are identified [39]. Following heparin treatment cessation, antibodies disappear from blood circulation within about 3 months. The respective concentrations of PF4 and heparin in blood circulation or at pathological sites are key factors for inducing immunogenicity [40, 41]. The clinical context is then a risk factor for heparin-dependent antibodies' development. Another initial cause which can favor generation of antibodies has been described and concerns a previous exposure of patients to bacterial infections [42]. PF4 can complex with bacterial polysaccharides and then becomes immunogenic. The immune response induces generation of antibodies to this chemokine. When patients with this former stimulation receive heparin, PF4 released from endothelium forms HPF4 complexes which reactivate the immune system (**Figure 1**), and IgG isotypes are rapidly generated. In addition to PF4, heparin treatment (and more especially LMWH) can also release tissue factor pathway inhibitor (TFPI) bound to ECs into blood circulation. No immune reaction to TFPI has been observed until now, but its increased concentration contributes to elevate the anticoagulant activity of heparin at the beginning of treatment.

4. Heparin-dependent antigens in HIT

The major heparin-dependent antigen involved in HIT/HITT is PF4, a CXC chemokine present in platelet α-granules and released upon platelet activation and aggregation. PF4 is a 70 amino acid (AA) protein with a MW of 7800 kDa, released in blood circulation as a tetramer with a MW of about 30 kDa [34–36, 43]. This chemokine has a structure involving one α-helix and three β-sheets organized in an antiparallel manner; it is highly electropositive, with many lysine and arginine residues, and has two disulfide bridges per monomer. The tetramer is organized in such a way that it exposes an external ring of positive charges, as shown in **Figure 3**. The formation of HPF4 complexes depends on the respective concentrations of heparin and PF4 [13, 24, 44]. Stoichiometric complexes are formed at a concentration of about 150 μg of heparin (i.e., about 27 IU UFH) per mg of PF4 (**Figure 4**). High- and low-affinity heparin molecules have the same reactivity with PF4, as well as LMWH, and the sulfation grade is of essence for these interactions. Patients who develop antibodies are those with the highest extracellular concentrations of PF4 in blood circulation, or at pathological sites, and with heparin concentrations permitting the formation of stoichiometric HPF4 complexes.

If heparin treatment is given through continuous infusion, heparin concentration remains constant in blood circulation, and the risk to form stoichiometric HPF4 reactive complexes is reduced. When heparin is given through the subcutaneous route, blood concentrations present high variations, from <0.1 IU/ml at trough to >0.7 IU/ml at peak. For current curative UFH treatments (2–3 injections/day),

DOI: http://dx.doi.org/10.5772/intechopen.86475

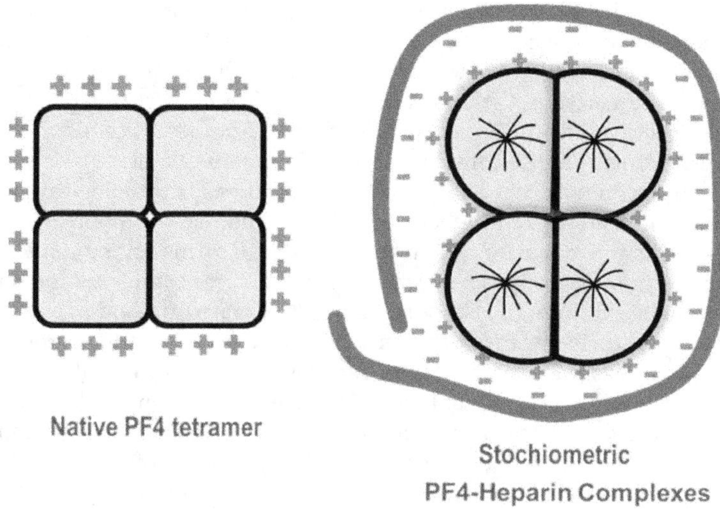

Figure 3.
Reaction of heparin with PF4 tetramers at stoichiometric concentrations. There is an intimate interaction between the ring of positive charges on the PF4 tetramer and the negative charges of the sulfated polysaccharide, heparin. This strong interaction induces an alteration of PF4 structure, rendering it immunogenic. Heparin (UFH or LMWH) molecules with at least 12 monosaccharides are required for this interaction.

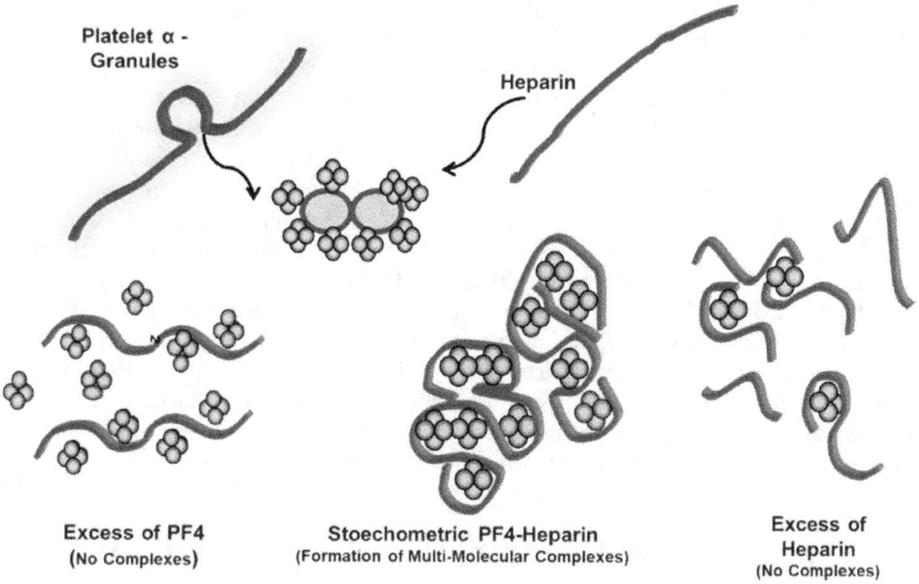

Figure 4.
PF4 is released from platelets as a complex with a proteoglycan dimer and is displaced by heparin for which it has a higher affinity. Complexes of heparin and PF4 depend on their respective ratios. When heparin and PF4 are at a stoichiometric concentration, large multimolecular complexes are formed and can be exposed on platelets or other blood cells. They can bind heparin-dependent antibodies and focus the deleterious immune reaction onto these cells. This can induce HIT or HITT in some patients.

the PF4 concentrations needed for forming stoichiometric complexes must be of about 4 μg/ml for heparin concentrations ≤0.1 IU/ml (trough) or of ≥28 μg/ml for heparin concentrations ≥0.7 IU/ml (peak). Required PF4 concentrations are high comparatively to expected heparin concentrations in blood circulation, even in disease states, but these high concentrations could be present at pathological sites. In ECC, blood heparin concentrations are high (about 4–5 IU/ml) and constant: formation of stoichiometric complexes can only occur with 25–30 µg/ml of PF4, which is unlikely. For information, the total amount of PF4 releasable from platelets, when they are totally activated and aggregated, is of about 5 µg per ml of blood (depending on platelet count and PF4 content; it is of ±12.5 ng/10^6 platelets).

But PF4 can accumulate and be at higher concentrations at pathological sites. Immunogenic stimulation occurs when body detects a non-self-component, which can be heparin used as anticoagulant. When bound to PF4, it forms large complexes, which can activate the immune response, which is targeted to these complexes and possibly extended to PF4 itself, through epitope spreading. Generated antibodies can be considered as alloantibodies. In few cases, PF4 antibodies can be pre-existing chronically or generated transitory as a side response to an infectious disease [14, 42, 45].
Anti-PF4 autoantibodies can bind to HPF4 complexes formed during heparin therapy and are then targeted to platelets or other blood cells which expose HPF4 complexes, focusing the deleterious immune response [22, 29, 30, 46]. In few cases, non-PF4 antigens can be involved [14, 15, 17, 46, 47]. HIT/HITT presentation and disease kinetics are then frequently atypical, although a moderate or characteristic thrombocytopenia develops during heparin therapy. IL8 has been reported in some patients as another heparin-dependent antigen in HIT/HITT. Anti-IL8 antibodies are pre-existing in many patients with chronic inflammation and are generated as a regulatory response to control this pathological context. Pathogenicity can occur because IL8 can bind heparin, and these complexes are fixed onto platelets and other blood cells through IL8 receptors (IL8-RA and IL8-RB) or through direct heparin binding [37, 38]. Interestingly, heparin binding to platelets increases with their activation grade. Anti-IL8 antibodies then focus the immune response deleterious effects to blood cells exposing heparin IL8 complexes which are then activated or destroyed. Neutrophil-activating peptide 2 (NAP-2), the β-thromboglobulin precursor, is another platelet CXC chemokine reported as a possible heparin-dependent antigen in rare HIT cases [14]. Lastly, in patients undergoing ECC [16, 26, 27], heparin is used as anticoagulant and is neutralized with a defined concentration of PrS at the end of the process. Anti-PrS or anti-heparin-PrS antibodies have been the only ones identified in few patients treated with heparin and presenting with a HIT-/HITT-like syndrome [17], with a possible fatal outcome. These antibodies can activate platelets in the presence of heparin [15, 46, 47]. Recent investigations have shown that anti-PrS antibodies are rather frequent in patients receiving this drug for heparin neutralization, but only very few of them develop severe clinical complications. Recurrent ECC in the same patient, with various exposures to heparin and PrS over time, can be an increased risk for development of antibodies and associated pathogenicity, with a HIT-/HITT-like syndrome.

5. Pathogenicity and mode of action of heparin-dependent antibodies

Heparin-dependent antibodies, and especially those to HPF4 complexes, induce thrombocytopenia and thrombosis in some clinical circumstances [46]. Particularly IgG isotypes can activate platelets, ECs, or other white blood cells such as monocytes, when they bind to their target antigenic structure, present at the surface of these cells [28, 29, 44, 46, 47]. There is now evidence that heparin and HPF4 complexes bind to platelets' surface, and this binding increases with their activation grade. HPF4 complexes fix antibodies and target the immune response, provoking platelet activation, aggregation, and interaction with other blood cells. During the process, IgGs react with platelet CD32, which is the FcγRIIa receptor [44, 46]. This contributes to amplify platelet activation and aggregation. The CD32 surface density is an important factor for the amplitude of platelet activation induced by antibodies. In patients with platelets presenting a CD32 polymorphism (131 Arg-His), activation is enhanced: the 131-Arg-His heterozygous or 131-His-His homozygous CD32 phenotypes are more reactive than the 131-Arg-Arg one. The patient propensity to develop HIT or HITT can depend on platelet activation grade and density or polymorphism of CD32. Antibodies to HPF4 can activate ECs and monocytes, favoring the release of TF, a potent procoagulant starter [29, 30]. In patients with HIT/HITT, neutrophils are activated and form aggregates with platelets, which can be detected in blood circulation. Therefore, the presence of anti-HPF4 IgG antibodies initiates multiple abnormal activities in blood circulation, which induce platelet activation and destruction and a concomitant prothrombotic risk (**Figure 5**). Blood activation can be out of control from body's antithrombotic defenses, which are overwhelmed, and thrombosis occurs. Interestingly, thrombosis tends to occur at pre-existing pathological sites, where blood activation and inflammation are already activated, and the risk is greatly amplified by anti-HPF4 antibodies, as summarized in **Figure 4**. We have the experience that an additional factor is very important for the initiation and amplification of the pathological process. This concerns the antibody avidity for HPF4 complexes [20]. In three patients with HIT or HITT, we succeeded to separate anti-HPF4 IgGs into two groups: the most important (>90%) one had a low affinity for HPF4 and no or only a weak platelet activation capacity, while the minor one (≤10%) activated highly platelets, as evidenced with the C_{14}-serotonin release assay. In few cases, only IgA isotypes specific for HPF4 complexes were identified in patients with HITT and malignant diseases. Although rare, IgAs can be pathogenic in some autoimmune disorders [49, 50], and this is not unexpected to note their effect in HIT. More rarely, IgM can be present at high concentration in patients with HIT, without IgGs. The mechanisms involved are not totally understood, but recently it was demonstrated that anti-HPF4 IgM antibodies can activate complement and induce platelet destruction [39]. Altogether, the different activities described here above help to understand why HPF4 antibodies, including IgG isotypes, can remain

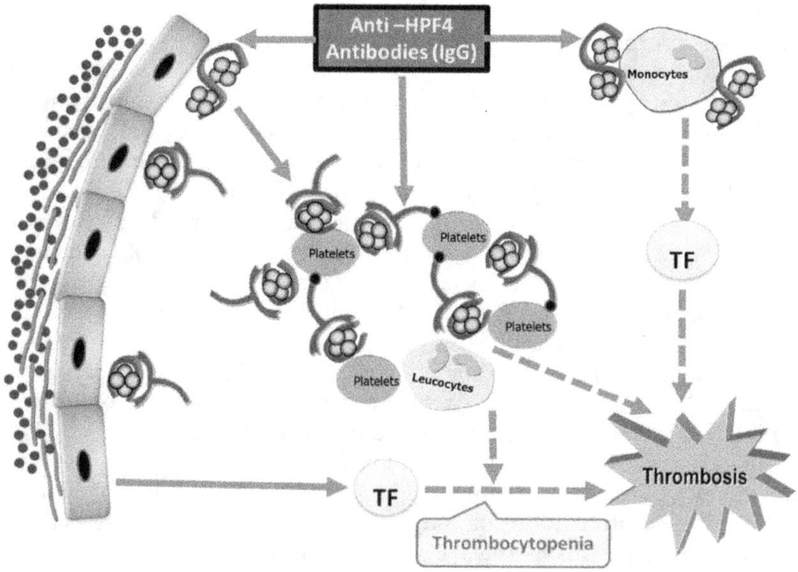

Figure 5.
Scheme showing how heparin-dependent antibodies, targeted to HPF4 complexes, bind to platelets and endothelial cells but also to monocytes and induce platelet and EC activation, monocyte stimulation, release of TF, and formation of aggregates, all contributing to thrombocytopenia and thrombosis.

asymptomatic in many patients and produce (especially IgG isotypes with high HPF4 affinity) HIT or HITT only in a few of them. The pathogenic process is multifactorial and involves activation and interaction of various blood cells, with the prothrombotic activity of TF. Patients' pathophysiological history and clinical status provide additional risk factors for the occurrence of disease [5, 6].

Nevertheless, there is still a fortuity context for the occurrence of the HIT/HITT complication, which relies on the formation of the immunoreactive HPF4 complexes, requiring defined concentrations of PF4 and heparin, exposed on blood cells [48]. This is a pre-requisite condition for permitting the binding of antibodies and starting the pathogenic process. This explains why this disease develops so rapidly when the critical conditions are met.

6. Diagnosis of heparin-induced thrombocytopenia

Many different assays are available for the diagnosis of heparin-dependent antibodies and for testing their capability to activate platelets. They are classified into two groups: immunoassays [23, 25, 51, 52], developed following the discovery of PF4 as the major target heparin-dependent antigen, and functional assays, performed with a low and a high heparin concentration, which were already used before [53]. A murine monoclonal antibody (KKO) has been developed and mimics HIT-associated antibodies, with platelet activation capability [54]. Here below we discuss the laboratory methods, and their combination, for the diagnosis of HIT/HITT. Diagnosis combines the clinical probability pretest with laboratory investigations [25]. For laboratory testing, the specimen used is plasma or serum for immunoassays and citrated plasma or heat-inactivated serum for functional assays. These techniques provide a laboratory support to establish, confirm, or exclude the diagnosis of HIT/HITT and must always be used in association with the pretest clinical probability. When HIT is suspected with a characteristic thrombocytopenia, heparin must be discontinued and replaced with another anticoagulant.

6.1 Immunoassays for heparin-dependent antibodies

With the discovery of the major target antigen for heparin-dependent antibodies, i.e., HPF4 complexes, immunoassays were developed, optimized, and standardized [23, 24, 52]. The first immunoassay introduced was a two-site enzyme-linked immunosorbent assay (ELISA), for measuring antibodies to HPF4 [12]. The antigen, HPF4, is coated on the plate, which is then saturated and stabilized. A well-defined stoichiometric concentration of PF4 tetramer and heparin (about 150 μg heparin per mg PF4) must be used for presenting epitopes reactive with antibodies. Heparin-dependent antibodies can be caught from the diluted tested plasma or serum (usually a 1:100 dilution is used), during the first incubation step. Following a washing step, the immunoconjugate, specific for human immunoglobulins or their isotypes, is introduced, and a second incubation step is performed. The immunoconjugate is often a rabbit or goat antibody, specific for human whole immunoglobulins (IgGAM) or for only an isotype (IgG, IgA, or IgM), and labeled with peroxidase. In current practice, this tag reagent is an antihuman IgG-peroxidase conjugate. Following a new washing step, the substrate is introduced, and a color develops. Tetramethylbenzidine (TMB) with hydrogen peroxide (H_2O_2) is now the most often used substrate, producing a blue color, which turns yellow when the reaction is stopped with sulfuric acid. Absorbance is measured using a microplate reader at 450 nm. Different variant methods have been introduced. Heparin can be replaced with another sulfated polymer (electronegative) such as polyvinyl sulfonate. However, using heparin matches better with the context of antibody generation and in vivo pathogenicity. Magnetic latex particles can be used in place of the solid phase capture micro-ELISA. Different tag antibody labels can be used instead of peroxidase, such as alkaline phosphatase (with its appropriate substrate). The "enzyme-substrate" detection system with chemiluminescence or fluorescence can also be used (direct measurement). Combining latex magnetic particles and chemiluminescence or fluorescence allows immunoassay automation. Lastly, performing immunoassays in the presence of an excess of heparin allows confirming antibody specificity [25, 55].

Figure 6 shows the general immunoassay principle for detecting heparin-dependent antibodies. For testing the non-PF4 antigen-dependent antibodies, similar immunoassays can be designed by replacing PF4 with the concerned protein (e.g., IL8 or PrS). We developed an original patented approach, where heparin in excess is coated in the presence of PrS and remains biologically available. The tested patient's sample is then incubated in the presence of a concentrated platelet lysate (containing all the platelet releasable proteins, but not plasma factors). If antibodies are present, a ternary complex is formed between tetrameric PF4 (or eventually another platelet protein), immobilized heparin, and antibodies. Caught antibodies are then detected as previously described [24]. This method offers a kinetic model for testing antibodies and mimics their binding to heparin-protein complexes bound onto platelet or blood cell surfaces. This assay reflects better the mechanisms occurring in pathology and offers improved and optimized sensitivity and specificity.

6.2 Platelet activation methods for disease confirmation

Functional assays rely on testing the capability of heparin-dependent antibodies to activate platelets at a low (0.1–1.0 IU/ml) and a high (10–100 IU/ml) heparin concentration. In HIT/HITT, platelets are only activated at the low heparin

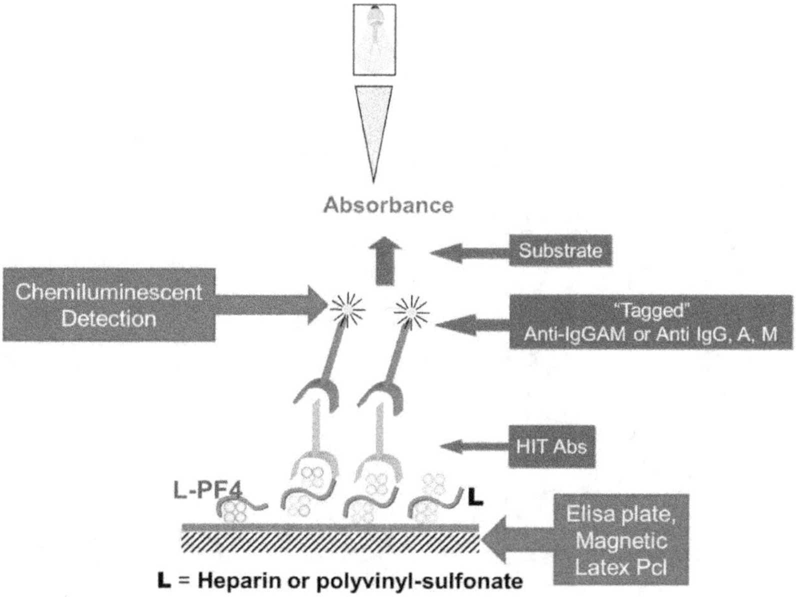

Figure 6.
General principle of immunoassays used for heparin-dependent antibodies, either globally or for specific isotypes. Enzyme tag with substrate is used in ELISA. Chemiluminescent immunoassays, using magnetic latex particles, can be automated on immunological analyzers. Using heparin in excess in sample diluent allows confirming antibody specificity.

concentration. Functional assays need to use normal donor platelets, freshly prepared. They must be duly selected for the right reactivity. This is the constraint which limits the use of this technique. Platelets are used as platelet-rich plasma (PRP) or as washed platelets. What induces donor to donor responsiveness in platelet activation assays used for HIT antibodies is not totally understood. The CD32 platelet density or His polymorphism could favor reactivity. In practice, platelets need to be qualified with a known positive sample for their appropriateness. Frequently, platelets from four normal donors are used, and the assay is positive if at least two out of the four donors give a positive platelet activation test. Other factors can regulate platelet activity, and interestingly washed platelets are usually more reactive than PRP. This can be explained by some platelet activation induced by the washing process, and a higher amount of PF4 is present on platelet surface. Functional assays concern PAT, SRA, heparin-induced platelet activation (HIPA), and flow cytometric assays (FCA); but other assays have been reported and elegantly reviewed in 2017 [53]. PAT is a simple aggregation assay performed with PRP and the tested patient citrated plasma. SRA is performed with washed platelets labeled with C_{14}, incubated with tested patient's plasma, and released C_{14}-serotonin is measured. HIPA is also performed with washed platelets, incubated with the tested sample, and platelet activation/aggregation is visually evaluated. FCA is a technique that requires to mix PRP (washed platelets are possible) with patient's citrated plasma and to measure platelet activation through the expression

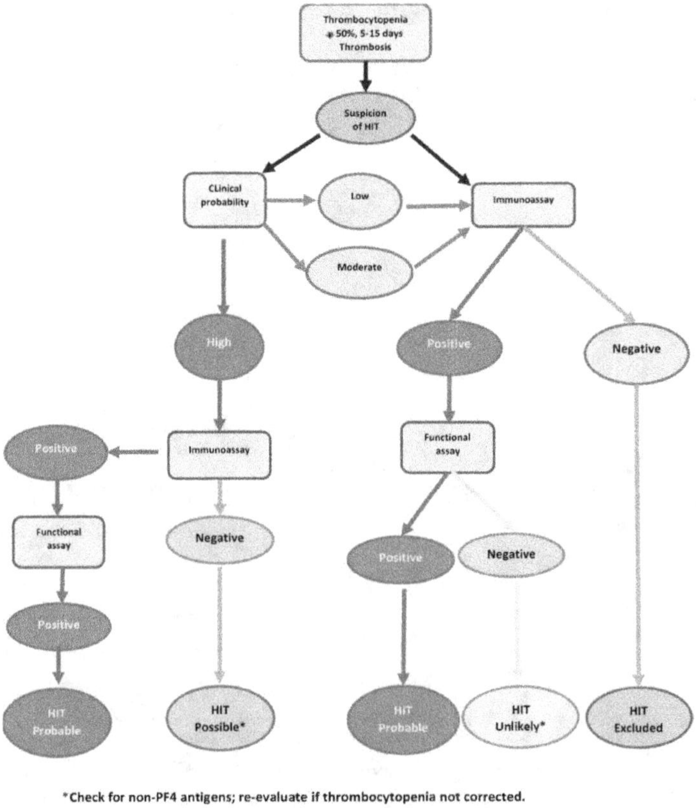

Figure 7.
Scheme showing the algorithm for the diagnosis of HIT/HITT: when suspected (thrombocytopenia and/or thrombosis), the disease diagnosis involves the clinical probability estimation and laboratory testing, first with immunoassay, which allows ruling out disease when not present, and then with a confirmatory functional assay.

of P-selectin [24]. FCA can also be used for the measurement of antibody-induced release of platelet microparticles. SRA is considered as the reference and most sensitive method. PAT has a poor sensitivity. HIPA needs trained laboratory operators and is mainly used in Germany and some neighboring countries. FCA is now a more standardized approach and looks promising but needs to be confirmed through practical experience in clinical laboratories. This method can be available in many centers for testing in emergency, provided a flow cytometer and fresh platelets are available.

6.3 Diagnostic approach for HIT/HITT

The diagnosis of HIT/HITT must be done accurately and reliably for a safe management of concerned patients [25]. The first alert signal is thrombocytopenia occurring 5–15 days following the onset of heparin therapy or earlier if the patient had a previous exposure to that drug within the 3 preceding months. HIT, or HITT if thrombosis is present, is then suspected and must rapidly be confirmed. If this complication is excluded, patients can continue to receive heparin, the most effective anticoagulant in many critical clinical situations. If the disease is confirmed or cannot be excluded, or if HIT is suspected but the diagnosis cannot be conducted, heparin must be replaced by another anticoagulant, according to the clinical context and practitioners' experience. **Figure** 7 shows an algorithm for establishing or excluding the diagnosis of HIT. When HIT is suspected, the pretest clinical probability must be evaluated with the 4Ts method or another one in use in the clinical setting [28]. The 4Ts score is simple and relatively well-standardized. When HIT/HITT is suspected, heparin is immediately stopped, and another anticoagulant is used to avoid any risk of severe complication. Nevertheless, the diagnosis must be established and confirmed, as the patient can need heparin later. The first laboratory investigation involves immunological testing for antibodies. If the test is negative, and the clinical probability is low or moderate, HIT can be excluded. But if clinical probability is high, HIT cannot be excluded and remains possible with non-PF4 heparin-dependent antigens involved. If positive, antibodies are present. HIT develops mainly when IgGs are generated and present at high concentration. Many authors consider that HIT occurs when the optical density (OD) in ELISA is >1.00 (the cutoff value for the positive range being at ≥0.5). When the IgG immunoassay is positive, a functional assay must be performed for confirming the diagnosis, as many heparin-dependent antibodies are asymptomatic. This functional assay must be as sensitive and specific as possible. In any case if clinical probability is high, the possibility of HIT complication remains present, whether the laboratory testing is. Testing must be repeated [56], and other antigens than HPF4 can be investigated.

7. Cross-reactivity of the various heparins, heparin-like compounds, or danaparoid sodium

HIT/HITT is associated with UFH or LMWH therapy, both drugs being sulfated polysaccharides. Other heparin-like anti-FXa anticoagulants, such as fondaparinux or danaparoid sodium, do not generate drug-specific antibodies [7, 10]. However, cross-reactivity of these drugs with antibodies present in patients with characterized HIT/HITT can be observed in laboratory assays [57]. This cross-reactivity has been reported for danaparoid sodium when it is tested in the immunoassay at a high concentration in the presence of PF4 (about 3.00 mg danaparoid sodium per mg of PF4). This can be due to the high-affinity heparan sulfate component present in this drug, which represents about 4% of the total. Cross-reactivity has also been reported in functional assays. However, there is no evidence that danaparoid sodium can generate drug-induced antibodies, and cross-reactivity is opposed by the other non-affinity components (about 80% low-affinity heparan sulfate, 12% dermatan sulfate, and 4% chondroitin sulfate), present in large excess, which disrupt the possible complexes formed, as do other low-sulfated polysaccharides [9, 58]. Therefore, there is no evidence that danaparoid sodium can provoke HIT/HITT, and the reported results and long-term clinical experience in many countries suggest that cross-reactivity is totally inhibited by the major non-affinity fractions. Furthermore, danaparoid sodium at therapeutic concentrations can inhibit the heparin-induced platelet aggregation. Conversely, pentosan polysulfate was found to be as effective as heparin and to form complexes with PF4 at similar ratios than UFH, for binding all heparin-dependent antibodies [8, 14]. Lastly, fondaparinux is not expected to induce drug-dependent antibodies or to cross-react with existing antibodies [32].

8. Conclusions and perspectives

In this chapter we have reviewed the present understanding of the generation of heparin-dependent antibodies in UFH- or LMWH-treated patients, which are the primary cause for HIT/HITT and a major adverse effect of heparin therapy. This risk is much higher when UFH is used, and disease develops more frequently in some clinical situations including cardiac or orthopedic surgery, traumatology, or malignancy. The occurrence of HIT/HITT tends to decrease thanks to a better control of therapy with UFH, shorter treatment times, and the use of LMWH when possible. When heparin therapy needs to be stopped, a large panel of alternative anticoagulants is available, although in some applications heparin remains the most effective one.

The mechanisms, which can induce generation of heparin-dependent antibodies, and pathogenicity for some of them have been extensively described and discussed in literature [14, 19, 20, 22, 42, 46]. Immunization develops when defined concentrations of heparin and PF4, forming stoichiometric multimolecular complexes, are present. In vivo, immunogenic complexes with PF4 can also be formed with other polyanions such as polyphosphates [59]. Various isotypes can be generated, IgM, IgA, or IgG, but almost all clinical complications of this iatrogenic disease are reported with IgGs present at high concentration and with high affinity. For HIT/HITT pathological development, various patient-associated and fortuity factors are required. Stoichiometric HPF4 complexes must be present for stimulating the immune system and developing antibodies but also for expressing pathogenicity. Heparin-dependent antibodies are harmful only if they bind to target antigenic structures (mainly HPF4 stoichiometric complexes), present on platelets, ECs, or other blood cells, focusing the immunological response. The immune system is then deviated from its protective role and destroys the patient's own cells [60].

HIT/HITT diagnosis is of essence for confirming or excluding this disease, and heparin treatment can be continued if the risk is ruled out. The first step when thrombocytopenia and/or thrombosis occur is to suspect this heparin adverse effect and to evaluate the pretest clinical probability. The 4Ts score is frequently used and allows risk classification from 0 to 8, 6–8 being the highest risk. Concomitantly, performing an immunoassay allows to detect and to measure IgG heparin-dependent antibodies targeted to HPF4. If the assay is negative and if clinical probability is low or moderate (score ≤ 5), HIT can be excluded, but patients need to be monitored closely, especially if thrombocytopenia is not corrected. If positive, IgG heparin-dependent antibodies are present, and HIT probability is higher if ELISA OD ≥ 1.00. Finally, the use of functional assays allows differentiating asymptomatic antibodies from those which can activate platelets and provoke disease. The presence of HIT or HITT is confirmed when the functional assay is positive [60]. However, even when negative, if clinical probability is high (6–8), HIT/HITT remains possible, and patients must be managed accordingly. Heparin cannot be continued in any patient with a possible or probable HIT diagnosis, and an alternative anticoagulant must be used.

Acknowledgements

The authors would like to thank the research groups with whom they had the opportunity and honor to collaborate and especially Profs. D. Meyer (Paris, France), A. Greinacher (Greifswald, Germany), T. Bakchoul (Tübingen, Germany), S. Panzer (Vienna, Austria), M. Poncz and G. Arepally (Philadelphia, USA), J. Fareed and J. Walenga (Chicago, USA), Y. Gruel and C. Pouplard (France), I. Elalamy (France), I. Gouin and P. Guéret (France), and all those who gave us the opportunity to investigate HIT.

Author details

Jean Amiral[1*] and Anne Marie Vissac[2]

1 Scientific-Hemostasis, Andresy, France

2 Hyphen-BioMed, Neuville sur Oise, France

*Address all correspondence to: jean.amiral@scientific-hemostasis.com

References

[1] Jang IK, Hursting MJ. When heparins promote thrombosis: Review of heparin-induced thrombocytopenia. Circulation. 2005;**111**:2671-2683

[2] Tardy-Poncet B, Piot M, Chapelle C, France G, Campos L, Garraud O, et al. Thrombin generation and heparin-induced thrombocytopenia. Journal of Thrombosis and Haemostasis. 2009;**7**:1474-1481

[3] Welsby IJ, Krakow EF, Heit JA, Williams EC, Arepally GM, Bar-Yosef S, et al. The association of anti-platelet factor 4/heparin antibodies with early and delayed thromboembolism after cardiac surgery. Journal of Thrombosis and Haemostasis. 2017;**15**:57-65

[4] Kuter DJ, Konkle BA, Hamza TH, Assmann LUSF, Kiss JE, Kaufman RM, et al. Clinical outcomes in a cohort of patients with heparin induced thrombocytopenia. American Journal of Hematology. 2017;**92**:730-738

[5] Dhakal B, Kreuziger LB, Rein L, Kleman A, Fraser R, Aster RH, et al. Disease burden, complication rates, and health-care costs of heparin-induced thrombocytopenia in the USA: A population-based study. Lancet Haematology. 2018;**5**(5):220-231

[6] Salter BS, Weiner MM, Trinh MA, Heller J, Evans AS, Adams DH, et al. Heparin-induced thrombocytopenia. A comprehensive clinical review. Journal of the American College of Cardiology. 2016;**67**(21):2519-2532

[7] Chong BH, Ismail F, Cade J, Gallus AS, Gordon S, Chesterman CN. Heparin-induced thrombocytopenia: Studies with a new low molecular weight heparinoid, Org 10172. Blood. 1989;**73**(6):1592-1506

[8] Greinacher A, Michels I, Mueller-Eckhardt C. Heparin-associated thrombocytopenia: The antibody is not heparin specific. Thrombosis and Haemostasis. 1992;**67**(5):545-549

[9] Krauel K, Hackbarth C, Fürll B, Greinacher A. Heparin-induced thrombocytopenia: In vitro studies on the interaction of dabigatran, rivaroxaban, and low-sulfated heparin, with platelet factor 4 and anti-PF4/heparin antibodies. Blood. 2012;**119**:1248-1255

[10] Kang M, Alahmadi M, Sawh S, Kovacs MJ, Lazo-Langner A. Fondaparinux for the treatment of suspected heparin-induced thrombocytopenia: A propensity score-matched study. Blood. 2015;**125**(6):924-929

[11] Nasiripour S, Saif M, Farasatinasab M, Emami S, Amouzegar A, Basi A, et al. Dabigatran as a treatment option for heparin-induced thrombocytopenia. Journal of Clinical Pharmacology. 2019;**59**(1):107-111

[12] Amiral J, Bridey F, Dreyfus M, Vissac AM, Fressinaud E, Wolf M, et al. Platelet factor 4 complexed to heparin is the target for antibodies generated in heparin-induced thrombocytopenia. Thrombosis and Haemostasis. 1992;**68**(1):95-96

[13] Amiral J, Bridey F, Wolf M, Boyer-Neumann C, Fressinaud E, Vissac AM, et al. Antibodies to macromolecular platelet factor 4-heparin complexes in heparin-induced thrombocytopenia: A study of 44 cases. Thrombosis and Haemostasis. 1995;**73**(1):21-28

[14] Amiral J, Marfaing-Koka A, Wolf M, Alessi MC, Tardy B, Boyer-Neumann C, et al. Presence of autoantibodies to interleukin-8 or neutrophil-activating peptide-2 in patients with heparin-associated thrombocytopenia. Blood. 1996;**88**(2):410-416

[15] Bakchoul T, Zöllner H, Amiral J, Panzer S, Selleng S, Kohlmann T, et al. Anti-protamine-heparin antibodies: Incidence, clinical relevance, and pathogenesis. Blood. 2013;**121**(15):2821-2827

[16] Lee GM, Welsby IJ, Phillips-Bute B, Ortel TL, Arepally GM. High incidence of antibodies to protamine and protamine/heparin complexes in patients undergoing cardiopulmonary bypass. Blood. 2013;**121**:2828-2835

[17] Panzer S, Schiferer A, Steinlechner B, Drouet L, Amiral J. Serological features of antibodies to protamine inducing thrombocytopenia and thrombosis. Clinical Chemistry and Laboratory Medicine. 2015;**53**(2):249-255

[18] Amiral J, Peynaud-Debayle E, Wolf M, Bridey F, Vissac AM, Meyer D. Generation of antibodies to heparin-PF4 complexes without thrombocytopenia in patients treated with unfractionated or low-molecular-weight heparin. American Journal of Hematology. 1996;**52**:90-95

[19] Greinacher A, Kohlmann T, Strobel U, Sheppard JAI, Warkentin TE. The temporal profile of the anti-PF4/heparin immune response. Blood. 2009;**113**(20):4970-4976

[20] Amiral J, Pouplard C, Vissac AM, Walenga JM, Jeske W, Gruel Y. Affinity purification of heparin-dependent antibodies to platelet factor 4 developed in heparin-induced thrombocytopenia: Biological characteristics and effects on platelet activation. British Journal of Haematology. 2000;**109**:336-341

[21] Rauova L, Poncz M, McKenzie SE, Reilly MP, Arepally G, Weisel JW, et al. Ultralarge complexes of PF4 and heparin are central to the pathogenesis of heparin-induced thrombocytopenia. Blood. 2005;**105**:131-138

[22] Rauova L, Zhai L, Kowalska MA, Arepally GM, Cines DB, Poncz M. Role of platelet surface PF4 antigenic complexes in heparin-induced thrombocytopenia pathogenesis: Diagnostic and therapeutic implications. Blood. 2006;**107**:2346-2353

[23] Bakchoul T, Giptner A, Bein G, Santoso S, Sachs UJH. Performance characteristics of two commercially available IgG-specific immunoassays in the assessment of heparin-induced thrombocytopenia (HIT). Thrombosis Research. 2011;**127**:345-348

[24] Amiral J, Seghatchian J. An update on evidence based diagnostic and confirmatory testing strategies for heparin induced thrombocytopenia using combined immunological and functional assays. Transfusion and Apheresis Science. 2018;**57**(6):804-811

[25] Favaloro EJ. Toward improved diagnosis of HIT. Blood. 2015;**126**:563-564

[26] Trossaërt M, Gaillard A, Commin PL, Amiral J, Vissac AM, Fressinaud E. High incidence of anti-heparin/platelet factor 4 antibodies cardiopulmonary bypass surgery. British Journal of Haematology. 1998;**101**:653-655

[27] Cuker A, Arepally GM, Chong BH, Cines DB, Greinacher A, Gruel Y, et al. Am Soc of Hemat 2018 guidelines for management of venous thromboembolism: Heparin-induced thrombocytopenia. Blood Advances. 2018;**2**(22):3360-3392

[28] Pouplard C, May MA, Iochmann S, Amiral J, Vissac AM, Marchand M, et al. Antibodies to platelet factor 4–heparin after cardiopulmonary bypass in patients anticoagulated with unfractionated heparin or a low-molecular-weight heparin clinical implications for heparin-induced

thrombocytopenia. Circulation. 1999;**99**:2530-2536

[29] Blank M, Shoenfeld Y, Tavor S, Praprotnik S, Boffa MC, Weksler B, et al. Anti-platelet factor 4/heparin antibodies from patients with heparin-induced thrombocytopenia provoke direct activation of microvascular endothelial cells. International Immunology. 2002;**14**(2):121-129

[30] Pouplard C, Iochmann S, Renard B, Herault O, Colombat P, Amiral J, et al. Induction of monocyte tissue factor expression by antibodies to heparin-platelet factor 4 complexes developed in heparin-induced thrombocytopenia. Blood. 2001;**97**(10):3300-3302

[31] Joglekar M, Khandelwal S, Cines DB, Poncz M, Rauova L, Arepally GM. Heparin enhances uptake of platelet factor 4/heparin complexes by monocytes and macrophage. Journal of Thrombosis and Haemostasis. 2015;**13**(8):1416-1422

[32] Amiral J, Lormeau JC, Marfaing-Koka A, Vissac AM, Wolf M, Boyer-Neumann C, et al. Absence of cross-reactivity of SR90107A/ORG31540 pentasaccharide with antibodies to heparin-PF4 complexes developed in heparin-induced thrombocytopenia. Blood Coagulation & Fibrinolysis. 1997;**8**:114-117

[33] Krauel K, Fürll B, Warkentin TE, Weitschies W, Kohlmann T, Sheppard JI, et al. Heparin-induced thrombocytopenia, therapeutic concentrations of danaparoid sodium, unlike fondaparinux and direct thrombin inhibitors, inhibit formation of platelet factor 4-heparin complexes. Journal of Thrombosis and Haemostasis. 2008;**6**(12):2160-2167

[34] Bock PE, Luscombe M, Marshall SE, Pepper DS, Holbrook JJ. The multiple complexes formed by the interaction of platelet factor 4 with heparin. The Biochemical Journal. 1980;**191**:769-776

[35] Denton J, Lane DA, Thunberg L, Slater AM, Lindhal U. Binding of platelet factor 4 to heparin oligosaccharides. The Biochemical Journal. 1983;**209**:455-460

[36] Mayo KH, Ilyna E, Roongta V, Dundas M, Joseph J, LAI MT, et al. Heparin binding to platelet factor-4 An NMR and site-directed mutagenesis study: Arginine residues are crucial for binding. The Biochemical Journal. 1995;**312**:357-365

[37] de Maistre E, Regnault V, Lecompte T, Scheid P, Martinet Y, Bellou A, et al. Antibodies to interleukin-8 and paraneoplastic catastrophic recurrent thrombosis. The American Journal of Medicine. 2001;**111**:580-581

[38] Regnault V, de Maistre E, Carteaux JP, Gruel Y, Nguyen P, Tardy B, et al. Platelet activation induced by human antibodies to interleukin-8. Blood. 2003;**101**(4):1419-1412

[39] Khandelwal S, Ravi J, Rauova L, Johnson A, Lee GM, Gilner JB, et al. Polyreactive IgM initiates complement activation by PF4/heparin complexes through the classical pathway. Blood. 2018;**132**(23):2431-2440

[40] Cai Z, Yarovoi SY, Zhu Z, Rauova L, Hayes V, Lebedeva T, et al. Atomic description of the immune complex involved in heparin-induced thrombocytopenia. Nature Communications. 2015;**22**(6):8277-8286

[41] Luna E, Agrawal P, Mehta R, Vernhes C, Viskov C, Amiral J, et al. Evaluation of immunostimulatory potential of branded and US-generic enoxaparins in an in vitro human immune system model. Clinical and Applied Thrombosis/Hemostasis. 2015;**21**(3):211-222

[42] Krauel K, Pötschke C, Weber C, Kessler W, Fürll B, Ittermann T, et al. Platelet factor 4 binds to bacteria,

inducing antibodies cross-reacting with the major antigen in heparin-induced thrombocytopenia. Blood. 2011;**117**:1370-1378

[43] Park KS, Rifat S, Eck H, Adachi K, Surrey S, Poncz M. Biologic and biochemic properties of recombinant platelet factor 4 demonstrate identity with the native protein. Blood Journal. 1990;**75**:1290-1295

[44] Suvarna S, Qi R, Arepally GM. Optimization of a murine immunization model for study of PF4/heparin antibodies. Journal of Thrombosis and Haemostasis. 2009;7:857-864

[45] Warkentin TE, Basciano PA, Knopman J, Bernstein RA. Spontaneous heparin-induced thrombocytopenia syndrome: 2 new, cases and a proposal for defining this disorder. Blood. 2014;**123**:3651-3654

[46] Newman PM, Chong BH. Heparin-induced thrombocytopenia: New evidence for the dynamic binding of purified anti-PF4-heparin antibodies to platelets and the resultant platelet activation. Blood. 2000;**96**:182-187

[47] BackchoulT JR, Warkentin TE. Protamine (heparin)-induced thrombocytopenia: A review of the serological and clinical features associated with anti-protamine/heparin antibodies. Journal of Thrombosis and Haemostasis. 2016;**14**:1685-1695

[48] Amiral J, Vissac AM. Role of heparin-dependent antigens in immune heparin-induced thrombocytopenia. In: HIT. 5th ed. London: CRC Press; 2012. DOI: 10.3109/9781841848617

[49] Aleyd E, Al M, Tuk CW, van der Laken CJ, van Egmond M. IgA complexes in plasma and synovial fluid of patients with rheumatoid arthritis induce neutrophil extracellular traps via FcαRI. Journal of Immunology. 2016;**197**(12):4552-4559

[50] Vavuli S, Salonurmi T, Loukovaara S, Nissinen AE, Savolainen MJ, Liinamaa MJ. Elevated levels of plasma IgA autoantibodies against oxidized LDL found in proliferative diabetic retinopathy but not in nonproliferative retinopathy. Journal Diabetes Research. 2016;**2016**:26141-26153

[51] Arepally G, Reynolds C, Tomaski A, Amiral J, Jawad A, Poncz M, et al. Comparison of PF4/heparin ELISA assay with the 14C-serotonin release assay in the diagnosis of heparin-induced thrombocytopenia. American Journal of Clinical Pathology. 1995;**104**:648-654

[52] Greinacher A, Potzsch B, Amiral J, Dummel V, Eichner A, Mueller-Eckhardt C. Heparin-associated thrombocytopenia: Isolation of the antibody and characterization of a multimolecular PF4-heparin complex as the major antigen. Thrombosis and Haemostasis. 1994;**71**(2):247-251

[53] Minet V, Dogné JM, Mullier F. Functional assays in the diagnosis of heparin-induced thrombocytopenia: A review. Molecules. 2017;**22**:617

[54] Arepally GM, Kamei S, Park KS, Kamei K, Li ZQ, Liu W, et al. Characterization of a murine monoclonal antibody that mimics heparin-induced thrombocytopenia antibodies. Blood. 2000;**95**:1533-1540

[55] Zheng G, Streiff MB, Takemoto CM, Bynum J, Gelwan E, Jani J, et al. The clinical utility of the heparin neutralization assay in the diagnosis of heparin-induced thrombocytopenia. Clinical and Applied Thrombosis/Hemostasis. 2018;**24**(5):749-754

[56] Omer T, Mullaguri N, George P, Newey CR. False-negative platelet factor 4 antibodies and serotonin release assay and the utility of repeat testing in the diagnosis of heparin-induced thrombocytopenia and

thrombosis, Hindawi case reports. Hematology. 2019;**2019**:1-4. DOI: 10.1155/2019/1585014

[57] Pouplard C, Amiral J, Borg JY, Vissac AM, Delahousse B, Gruel Y. Differences in specificity of heparin-dependent antibodies developed in heparin-induced thrombocytopenia and consequences on cross-reactivity with danaparoid sodium. British Journal of Haematology. 1997;**99**:273-280

[58] Joglekar MA, Quintana Diez PM, Marcus S, Qi R, Espinasse B, Wiesner MR, et al. Disruption of PF4/H multimolecular complex formation with a minimally anticoagulant heparin (ODSH). Thrombosis and Haemostasis. 2012;**107**:717-725

[59] Cines DB, Yarovoi SV, Zaitsev SV, Lebedeva T, Rauova L, Poncz M, et al. Polyphosphate/platelet factor 4 complexes can mediate heparin-independent platelet activation in heparin-induced thrombocytopenia. Blood Advances. 2016;**1**(1):62-74

[60] Greinacher A. Heparin induced thrombocytopenia. The New England Journal of Medicine. 2015;**373**:252-261

Chapter 4

Examination of Laboratory for Monitoring Heparin Anticoagulant Therapy

Yetti Hernaningsih and Ersa Bayung Maulidan

Abstract

Heparin-derivative anticoagulants include unfractionated heparin (UFH), low molecular weight heparin (LMWH), pentasaccharide (fondaparinux), and ultralow molecular weight heparin (ULMWH). Heparin contains an active pentasaccharide sequence that binds to antithrombin (AT). This bond produces conformational changes that accelerate its binding with AT and inactivation of coagulation factors XIIa, XIa, Xa, and IXa and thrombin (IIa). Thrombin and factor Xa are the most sensitive to inhibition by the heparin-AT complex, and the strength of inhibiting thrombin is ten times more sensitive than factor Xa. The UFH anticoagulant response is monitored using activated partial thromboplastin time (APTT), a measurement that is sensitive to inhibition of thrombin and factor Xa. Protamine titration examination is the standard for measuring UFH concentrations in plasma. Recommendations from the American College of Chest Physicians (ACCP) suggest that the APTT target range for the UFH therapy is equivalent to 0.2–0.4 IU/mL with protamine titration or 0.35–0.7 IU/mL with an anti-Xa examination. A new examination is thrombodynamics (TD), measuring the level of development of clots. This method is considered most able to mimic the coagulation process that occurs in vivo compared to other examinations.

Keywords: heparin, anticoagulant, PPT, APTT, anti-Xa, protamine, thrombodynamics

1. Introduction

At present the use of anticoagulants is very wide; about 0.7% of the population in the west receives anticoagulant treatment. Basic anticoagulant therapy is a vitamin K antagonist; a derivative of warfarin, which is most commonly used, is coumadin (warfarin). This drug has been used for more than 50 years and is consistently able to eliminate recurrent venous thrombosis at adequate doses. However, warfarin has disadvantages, namely, the interaction with other drugs and with food, slow onset and excessive effects, and a narrow therapeutic range. Drug responses and pharmacodynamics are varied and unpredictable, so routine monitoring is needed. For most patients who take drugs in the long term, this is quite troublesome [1].

The current world medical need is to find anticoagulants that are more effective and safer than warfarin for both doctors and patients in long-term use. Responding to this need, a new drug is needed that can change molecules that are difficult to absorb to be easily absorbed through the digestive tract; this is used as the basis for making oral preparations of unfractionated heparin (UFH). In theory the use of the oral form of heparin or low molecular weight heparin (LMWH) is given at fixed doses, two or three times a day, and does not require overly frequent coagulation monitoring checks or dosage adjustments which are too tight, and the potential for interactions between drugs and medications is also low, making this drug an anticoagulant needed for long-term use [1].

Coagulation monitoring for patients receiving heparin therapy is very important. This is intended to obtain a range of heparin therapy that is effective in reducing the incidence of thrombus and bleeding. The effective use of heparin anticoagulant therapy must increase the activated partial thromboplastin time (APTT) value from 1.5 to 2.5 times. This value is equivalent to levels of heparin 0.2–0.4 U/mL based on protamine titration and is equivalent to anti-Xa levels 0.3–0.7 U/mL [2]. This chapter will discuss laboratory tests that are used to monitor patients receiving heparin therapy.

2. Development of heparin

Heparin is the oldest anticoagulant used in medicine. Heparin was discovered by McLean in 1916 while trying to isolate thromboplastic agents. Heparin is a polysaccharide from the class of glycosaminoglycans (GAG) which naturally appears on all mast cells. Further research in 1935 resulted in clinical use of heparin. Since then, heparin has been widely studied for various applications and modifications [3].

Unfractionated heparin (UFH) is a product of GAG purified from animal tissue, most often from pig intestines. Heparin provides indirect anticoagulant properties by binding to antithrombin III (ATIII) and facilitating the inhibitory effects possessed by AT on thrombin and activated X factor (factor Xa). It is known that only UFH contains at least 18 saccharide sequences that can affect AT activity and thrombin, whereas UFH with a series of certain pentasaccharides can inhibit the activity of factor Xa [3] (**Figure 1**).

The heterogeneity of the structure of the UFH causes extensive bioactivity and physiological activity. Some heparin chains bind to other plasma proteins and have an effect on bone metabolism resulting in osteoporosis or heparin-induced thrombocytopenia (HIT) and other unpredictable effects that require continuous monitoring. Further research and discoveries resulted in low molecular weight heparins (LMWH) in the late 1970s to early 1980s; this was to find anticoagulants which were more predictable in their activities [4]. LMWH, such as enoxaparin, dalteparin, and tinzaparin, is made by chemical control or enzymatic cutting of UFH in a depolymerization reaction.

This controlled process produces fragments with lower molecular weight and more predictable action than UFH. As a result, side effects are lighter than UFH, monitoring needs are decreased, and bioavailability increases, making LMWH potentially used for outpatients. This makes LMWH the standard of care replacing UFH except in certain cases such as kidney failure and acute coronary syndrome where UFH is still preferred because the liver clearance is lighter and better reversible with protamine sulfate [5].

Ultralow molecular weight heparin (ULMWH) was discovered in early 2000 through a process of chemical synthesis. The reason is to get agents with lighter side effects but have the same or better anticoagulant effect which causes a higher anti-factor Xa ratio to antithrombin activity [6].

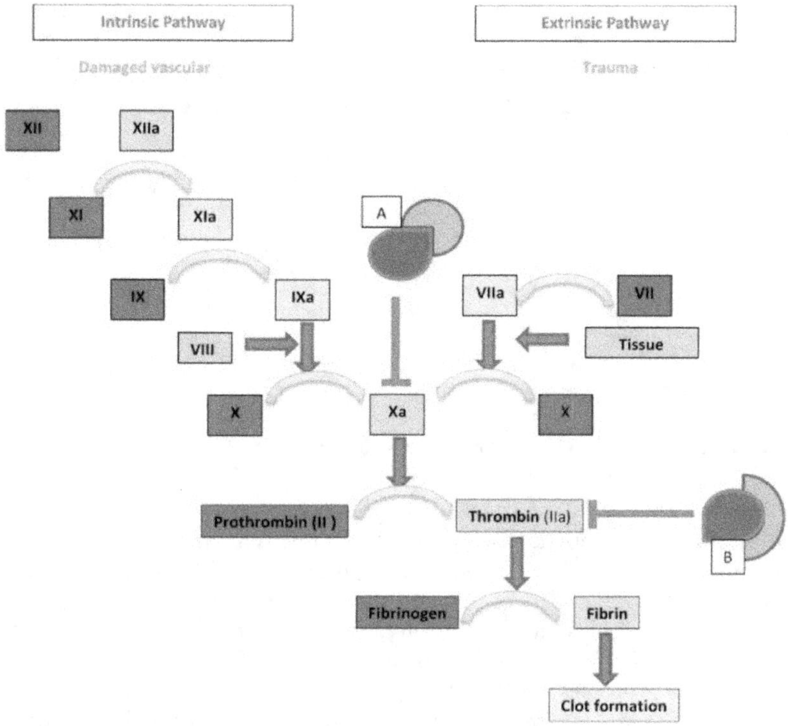

Figure 1.
Mechanism of heparin in the coagulation cascade. Box A: AT (red) binds to a heparin fragment (green) with any series length provided that certain pentasaccharide bonds can inhibit factor Xa. Box B: AT (red) binds to heparin (green) with a chain length > 17 U of disaccharide that can inhibit thrombin (factor IIa) [3].

3. Structure and biosynthesis of heparin

Heparin is a polydisperse and highly sulfated GAG with a molecular weight between 5 and 40 kDa. The structure of the complex contains repetitive disaccharide units that contain uronic acid residues (L-iduronic (IdoA) or D-glucuronic acid (GlcA)) and N-acetyl-D-glucosamine. The biosynthesis process of heparin starts in the endoplasmic reticulum and the Golgi apparatus of mast cells. The tetrasaccharide link attaches to the residue of serine in the core protein, serglycin, and then adds a unit of D-glucuronic acid (1→4) N-acetyl-D-glucosamine disaccharide. Disaccharide sulfonation and epimerization of glucoronate to iduronate are carried out by various enzymes in the biosynthetic pathway. In total there are 12 enzymes involved in this pathway, which act together to form the desired molecule. These involved enzymes have many isoforms, which cause heterogeneity of heparin and allow these enzymes to directly biosynthesize associated GAG, heparin sulfate. The degree of sulfation and sulfate residue allocation depends on the spectrum of activity of the product. In mast cell degradation, peptidoglycan heparin changes to GAG heparin through protease and β-endo glucuronidase activity [3].

The first glycosaminoglycan-protein bonding region is formed due to glycotransferase activity. Repeated disaccharide units undergo elongation by GlcA and GLcNAc transferase. Modified chains include N-deacetylation and N-sulfonation, O-sulfonation, and epimerization, which then occur due to specific enzyme activity. The monosaccharide symbol in this figure follows the symbol nomenclature for glycan (SFNG) system [3] (**Figure 2**).

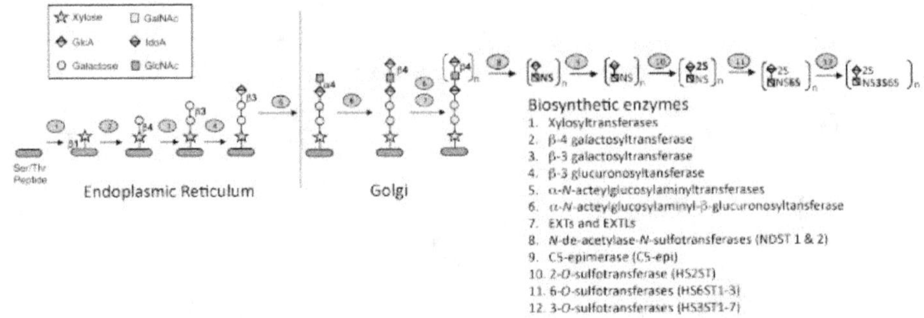

Figure 2.
Heparin biosynthesis.

4. Mechanism of heparin as an anticoagulant

Heparin has anticoagulant effects through interactions with coagulation factors and inhibitors. Coagulation is a complex process involving proteins, platelets, and cellular components such as endothelium and monocytes. The balance of hemostasis is maintained if the activity of procoagulant can be balanced with an inhibitor. The main inhibitor of plasma coagulation factor is AT, which acts on active coagulation factors such as FXIIa, FXIa, FXa, FIXa, FVIIa, and FIIa. These coagulation factors are serine proteases, so AT is a serine protease inhibitor (serpin).

Heparin, acting as a catalyst, provides anticoagulation activity by potentiating other AT and serpin inhibitor activities (**Figure 3**). The interaction of heparin with AT requires a certain sequence of pentasaccharides, but not so with other serpins.

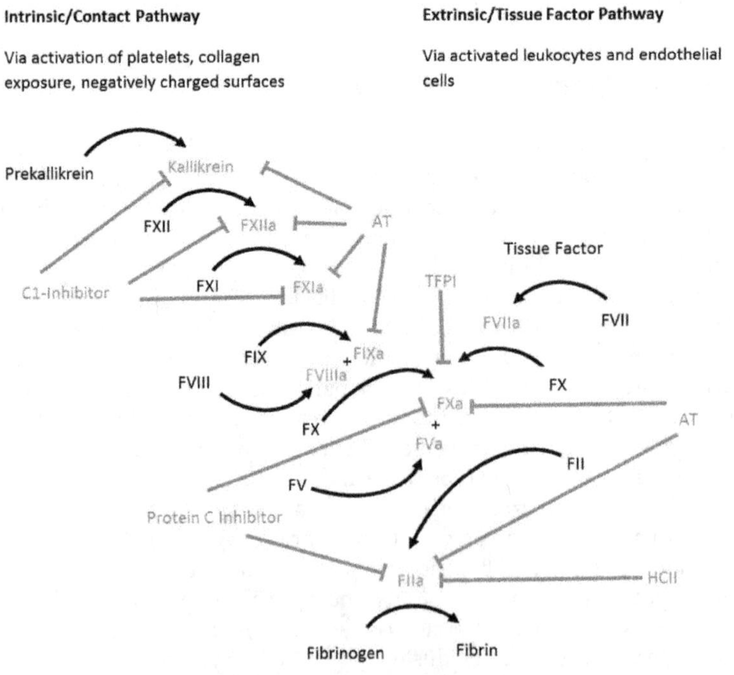

Figure 3.
Interaction of the coagulation factor with serpin. The blue line shows the place of inhibition of each serpin [11]. TFPI, tissue factor pathway inhibitor; AT, antithrombin; HCII, heparin cofactor II.

Another important heparin-binding inhibitor on the extrinsic pathway is tissue factor pathway inhibitors (TFPI) [7–9].

Antithrombin (AT) under conditions when it does not bind to heparin is a slow-acting serpin, because the reactive center loop is partially folded to the center of the b-sheet structure. When binding to heparin, AT inhibition activity will increase significantly, which is a characteristic of serpin. The high-affinity pentasaccharides in heparin bind to antithrombin through two stages: first, the initial binding process involves three monosaccharide units and initiates conformational changes to AT, and then after the interaction is complete, AT conformation after activation by heparin is stabilized. This conformational change is transmitted to the AT structure, causing the opening of the reactive center loop and an increase in exosite exposure from AT which binds directly to FXa [10].

4.1 Inhibition of antithrombin in factors IIa and Xa

Active AT conformation caused by pentasaccharides is sufficient to increase inhibitory activity in FXa, a protease that converts prothrombin to thrombin (FIIa). Factor Xa interacts directly with AT in specific exosite exposed when binding to heparin. In addition, in the presence of calcium, a single heparin chain can bind directly to AT and FXa, increasing AT-FXa interactions, but this is not absolutely necessary. This calcium-dependent effect can account for reports of calcium-induced-specific molecules during the FXa inhibition process by AT [12]. Heparin-mediated FXa binds to AT, indicating the longer heparin chain will increase its affinity with the presence of Ca^{2+} and will strengthen inhibition [13].

Unlike FXa, the potentiation of thrombin inhibition by AT requires an additional 13 saccharide chains attached to the nonreductive end of the pentasaccharide sequence, so thrombin and AT are bound to the same heparin molecule. Thrombin interacts with heparin in exosite II, which is basically a different method with AT; no specific heparin is needed for this interaction [14].

4.2 Inhibition of antithrombin in other coagulation factors

Antithrombin also inhibits several other protease coagulant factors. The way antithrombin blocks FIXa is similar to FXa, which binds to the same exosite on AT. The high-resolution crystal structure of the pentasaccharide-FIXa-AT complex shows that one pentasaccharide binds to AT and the second binds to exosite from FXa, which allows a relationship between the two proteins with one molecule of heparin [13].

The ability of heparin to increase AT inhibition in FXI and kallikrein in the intrinsic coagulation pathway is relatively limited compared to FXa and thrombin. It should be noted that FXI activity in AT mutants that bind to the heparin site is still slightly potentiated by heparin, suggesting that there is a direct interaction between heparin and FXI involved in the binding sites of potential heparin found in the FXI catalytic domain [11].

Antithrombin inhibits the FVIIa complex in the extrinsic pathway, and this effect is reinforced by fondaparinux, LMWH, and UFH. Direct and calcium-dependent interactions are found between FVIIa and heparin [11].

4.3 Other serpins activated by heparin

Heparin cofactor II (HCII), another serpin potentiated by heparin, is a coagulation inhibitor that only inhibits thrombin. HCII is also reported to inhibit chymotrypsin and neutrophil cathepsin G. Heparin cofactor II is found in plasma at the same level as AT, but HCII cannot replace AT if there is a deficiency. HCII deficiency has no effect on the coagulation system but results in increased formation of an occlusive arterial thrombus after endothelial damage. In vivo HCII is potentiated by dermatan sulfate, which is found in the walls of blood vessels. HCII activated by dermatan sulfate may play a role in preventing excessive thrombosis of injured blood vessels [15].

Heparin and dermatan sulfate both potentiate inhibition of thrombin through HCII in several stages. Unlike AT, HCII does not require a certain series of heparin to interact. Other polyanions can also bind to HCII. The HCII bond with heparin causes conformational changes similar to AT while also releasing thrombin-binding N-terminal tail. The combination of reactive center loop expulsion initiated by GAG by exposure to exosite protease-binding is controlled by AT and HCII in the opposite way [16, 17].

Protein C inhibitors (PCI) regulate the activity of activated protein C (APC), which is the active form of zymogen protein C. Protein C is converted to APC by thrombin and in its active form acts as an anticoagulant by inactivating FVa and FVIIIa, in the presence of protein cofactors S. PCI regulates coagulation inhibitors, in this case acting more as a supporter of coagulation than inhibiting coagulation. The bond of heparin to PCI strengthens the inhibition of APC and FXa in the presence of calcium. A long chain of heparin is needed to strengthen APC inhibition, which suggests both PCI and protease require simultaneous bonding with heparin. The basic structure of the PCI complex with heparin and thrombin if separated, binding sites for heparin will appear involving the H helix, which is located close to the reactive loop [18].

The importance of protease nexin (PN)-1 in the last biology and hemostasis is known. In vitro serpin is known to have an effect of approximately 100 times faster than AT, and heparin increases about 3 times. In vivo PN-1 does not contribute to the activity of heparin as an anticoagulant because its concentration in plasma is very low; on the contrary, PN-1 is found to bind to the cell surface in several organs and tissues, including blood vessel walls. Protease nexin (PN)-1 is detected in platelet granules on the platelet surface and secreted during platelet activation. In this context, the contribution of PN-1 to antithrombotic activity from heparin in vivo is ignored [19].

The crystal structure of PN-1 is obtained from the breakdown of complexes with heparin and thrombin. This protein has a typical serpin fold with the heparin-binding site in helix D. Contrary to AT, heparin-binding site PN-1 and thrombin are not parallel when the reactive center loop of PN-1 productively interacts with the active part of thrombin. The initial formation of the ternary complex between PN-1 and thrombin and heparin can be said to be the initial phase of two-phase interaction, with loss of heparin-thrombin interactions when covalent complex PN-1 thrombin is formed. Heparin is not released when forming the PN-1-thrombin complex; this shows that the PN-1-thrombin complex is still bound to HS on the cell surface [11, 20].

Protein Z-dependent proteinase inhibitors are known to inhibit both FXa and FXIa. Heparin speeds up this reaction 20–100×. The heparin-binding site on protein Z-dependent protease inhibitors involves basic residues in helix D (such as AT) and helix C (unlike AT), and the presence of unstructured N-terminal ends can indicate similarities with HCII [21].

Other serpins, c1inh, inhibit both the complement cascade and the intrinsic pathway, where the coagulation system and innate immune system interact. Clinical deficiency leads to congenital angioedema through excessive contact system activity. The effects of c1inh are not limited to complement and contact systems. Heparin potentiates the activity of the c1inh, and the crystal structure of the c1inh indicates a different model of activity against different protease and heparin-binding sites against AT [22].

4.4 Non-serpin inhibitors: tissue factor pathway inhibitors

Tissue factor pathway inhibitors (TFPI) are structurally serpin, but not serine protease inhibitors. Tissue factor pathway inhibitors (TFPI) are major inhibitors in the extrinsic pathway. The heparin-binding TFPIα isoform contains an acidic N-terminal region, three Kunitz domain pairs, and a basic C-terminal end. Kunitz domain is involved in anticoagulant activity, with the first domain inhibiting the FVIIa-tissue factor complex and the second domain inhibiting FXa. The C-terminal circuit in TFPI has a high affinity for heparin. Heparin injection releases TFPI bound to the endothelium to the circulation. Heparin bound to TFPI potentiates inhibitory activity in both free FXa and FXa in the FVIIa-TF-FXa complex [11].

5. The drug derivate heparin

5.1 Unfractionated heparin

Unfractionated heparin (UFH) is one of the most commonly used parenteral anticoagulants to treat or prevent thromboembolism and has been used for almost a century. This drug is used in various methods, such as systemic use, through a catheter, extracorporeal, or on the surface of a medical device to prevent thrombotic complications. Heparin depends on the presence of antithrombin (AT) to inhibit clotting factors, so heparin is called an anticoagulant which acts indirectly. Heparin does not have fibrinolytic activity and will not lyse the thrombus [23].

Heparin contains an active pentasaccharide sequence that binds AT. The active pentasaccharide sequence responsible for catalyzing AT is found in one third and one tenth of the UFH and LMWH chains. After heparin binds and activates AT, heparin can release AT and bind other ATs, thus providing a continuous anticoagulant effect. This bond produces conformational changes that accelerate binding of AT and inactivation of coagulation factors XIIa, XIa, Xa, and IXa and thrombin (IIa). Thrombin and factor Xa are the most sensitive to inhibition by the heparin/AT, and tenfold thrombin complex is more sensitive to inhibition than factor Xa [23, 24].

The inhibition of UFH on thrombin requires binding of coagulation enzymes and AT through high-affinity pentasaccharides, whereas inhibition of factor Xa requires only heparin binding to AT. By deactivating thrombin, heparin not only prevents fibrin formation but also inhibits platelet activation induced by thrombin and coagulation factors V and VIII. In addition to its anticoagulation effects, heparin increases the permeability of blood vessel walls, suppresses smooth muscle proliferation, suppresses osteoblast formation, and activates osteoclasts [23, 24].

5.1.1 Pharmacokinetics and pharmacodynamics

Intravenous (IV) or subcutaneous (SC) injection is the route available for UFH administration, and IV is the most frequently used route. When given by SC injection for therapeutic anticoagulation, the dose must be large enough (30,000 U/day) to compensate for the low bioavailability of UFH, as can be seen in **Table 1**. UFH is already bound to plasma proteins, which results in variations in anticoagulant responses [25].

Characteristics	Heparin	LMWH
Origin	Pig intestine	Pig intestine
Molecular weight (Da)	15,000	5000
Target	Xa:IIa	Xa > IIa
Bioavailability (%)	30	90
Half-life (h)[a]	IV depends on doses 1–3	3–7
	SC depends on doses 2–5	
Reversal by protamine	Complete	Partial (60–80%)
Renal excretion	Depends on dose	Yes
Occurrence of heparin-induced thrombocytopenia (%)	<5.0	<1.0

[a] *In normal renal function.*

Table 1.
Pharmacological properties of UFH and LMWH [26].

UFH clearance depends on the dose and occurs through two independent mechanisms. The initial phase is a fast and saturated bond in endothelial cells, macrophages, and local proteins where UFH is depolymerized. The second phase is slower and unsaturated clearance through the kidneys. At therapeutic doses, UFH is cleared mainly through depolymerization, where higher molecular weight chains are cleared faster than those with lower weight. When clearance tends to the kidneys, an increase or extension of the dose of UFH provides a disproportionate increase in both the intensity and duration of the anticoagulant effect. Anticoagulant responses to UFH administration are usually monitored using activated partial thromboplastin time (APTT). APTT must be measured every 6 hours with IV administration and the dose adjusted until the patient has reached a stable level of therapy. After a stable condition is reached, the frequency of monitoring can be extended [24, 26].

5.1.2 Monitoring

The UFH anticoagulant response is monitored using APTT, a measurement that is sensitive to inhibition of thrombin and FXa. APTT examinations have a large variety of reagents (even the same reagents have different lots) so that they have varying sensitivity to the anticoagulant effect of UFH. Each laboratory must ensure that their therapeutic range of heparin and APTT is based on levels of heparin measured by anti-Xa (target range 0.3–0.7 U/mL) or protamine titration (0.2–0.4 U/mL). APTT must be measured every 6 h based on UFH half-life and the dose adjusted until the patient reaches the therapeutic level based on the APTT target range. When APTT values are obtained in the treatment range twice in a row, monitoring can be extended to one or two times a day depending on the clinical scenario. Weight-based dose nomograms, consisting of bolus doses and infusion droplet speeds with regular monitoring using APTT, are recommended for the treatment of thromboembolic disease [25].

The UFH dose nomogram differs in each hospital due to differences in thromboplastin reagents, calibration, and interlaboratory standards in APTT measurements. This causes the need for alternative monitoring methods. Functional heparin, also known as anti-Xa, has been promoted as a more reliable measure of UFH because it is not sensitive to factors other than UFH, such as concomitant use of warfarin, sodium citrate in the sample tube, impaired lupus anticoagulant (LA), increased factor activity VIII, and liver disease [25].

Acquired inhibitors, such as LA, cause an extension of APTT, which results in not being able to accurately measure the level of anticoagulation due to UFH.

In this case, if APTT is maintained within the usual therapeutic range, it may result in underdose of UFH and cause development or recurrence of thrombosis. Simultaneous testing of APTT and anti-Xa levels is needed to estimate the APTT value of therapy in patients receiving heparin [27].

5.2 Low molecular weight heparin (LMWH)

LMWH is a polysaccharide derived from the pig's intestine containing an active pentasaccharide sequence which is needed for anticoagulant activity as in UFH. LMWH is produced from UFH through chemical or enzymatic degradation. Each LMWH product is prepared by a different method. Clinical development of LMWH driven by certain observations includes the reduction of thrombin activity in relation to anti-factor Xa activity, the ratio of benefits or risks that are more favorable in animal studies, and good pharmacokinetic properties. The molecular weight of the LMWH is approximately one third of the molecular weight of UFH (4000–5000 Da). Because of their smaller size, LMWH has a lower affinity for thrombin because they cannot bind AT and thrombin together. However, LMWH has the same affinity as UFH for FXa [23].

Factor Xa does not require heparin to stabilize its interaction with AT, so smaller molecules such as LMWH deactivate factor Xa equivalent to larger molecules such as UFH. The length of the polysaccharide chain of at least 18 saccharides, including the order of active pentasaccharides, is needed to bridge between AT and thrombin. About 25–50% of LMWH molecules are above the length of this chain. All LMWH chains contain active pentasaccharide sequences, so 100% can inactivate factor Xa [23].

5.2.1 Pharmacodynamics and pharmacokinetics

There are several biological consequences of the small size of LMWH compared to UFH, a decrease in binding of LMWH to other plasma proteins, macrophages, and endothelial cells. This resulted in a more predictable dose-response relationship and a longer plasma half-life for LMWH. In contrast to UFH, routine plasma monitoring is not needed which makes it easier for outpatient management. The lower incidence of HIT has also been investigated because of the reduced bond to PF4 and platelets. LMWH has also reduced bonds in osteoblasts resulting in decreased incidence of osteoclast activation and lower bone destruction [23].

All LMWH products have half-lives ranging from 3 to 7 h and bioavailability 87–90%. Anti-Xa peak activity occurs 3–5 h after SC injection with predictable dose-based responses. All agents are metabolized through desulfation or depolymerization, and all agents metabolized are excreted through the kidneys [25].

5.3 Pentasaccharides (fondaparinux)

Fondaparinux is a chemically synthesized anticoagulant that is specifically developed as a selective indirect inhibitor for FXa. Factor Xa is an important target for anticoagulant therapy given its position at the meeting of the intrinsic and extrinsic coagulation pathways. Its inhibition significantly decreases thrombin formation [28] (**Figure 4**).

Factor Xa has one function in the coagulation cascade, as a gatekeeper to the path along the coagulation cascade. Conversely, thrombin (FIIa) has many roles in the coagulation process, including activation and mediation of endogenous anticoagulation by binding to thrombomodulin and activation of protein C. Factor Xa may be a purer target than thrombin [29].

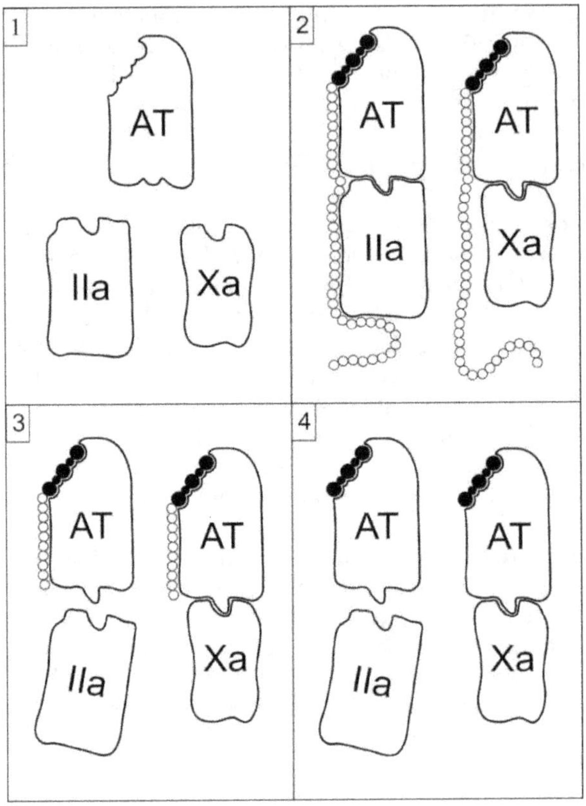

Figure 4.
Formation of antithrombin complexes with FIIa and FXa. (1) Antithrombin (AT), active thrombin (FIIa), active X factor (FXa). (2) UFH (chain shape) forms a complex with AT both in FIIa and FXa. (3) Shorter polysaccharides of 18 U form AT complex with FXa but not with FIIa. (4) The sequence of pentasaccharides forms a bond with FXa only [30].

5.3.1 Pharmacodynamics and pharmacokinetics

Fondaparinux binds non-covalently and reversibly to AT, increasing AT anticoagulant activity by up to 300 times. The AT-fondaparinux complex then binds and neutralizes FXa, which reduces prothrombin (FII) conversion to thrombin (FIIa), thereby inhibiting clot formation. Fondaparinux is then released and can catalyze other AT molecules. When AT plasma becomes saturated, excess unbound circulating fondaparinux (which has no anticoagulant activity) is excreted through the kidneys.

Because it does not affect pre-existing thrombin circulation, fondaparinux may in theory have some residual hemostatics, if needed, at the site of injury. Fondaparinux has no effect on the examination of fibrinogen platelet function, thrombin time, or antithrombin tests. Fondaparinux can affect PT and APTT and can interfere with factor VIII testing. Although not routinely recommended, if measurements of fondaparinux are needed (e.g., changes in kidney function, weight, or extreme age), the most accurate plasma concentration is measured using the anti-factor Xa test. The results of this examination are in IU/mL, which is directly proportional to the plasma concentration of fondaparinux. The results were extrapolated to the mcg/mL plasma concentration using a standard curve calibrated by fondaparinux. The test must be calibrated specifically for fondaparinux, because the use of calibration for UFH or LMWH will produce inaccurate results.

The use of fondaparinux and drugs that affect concomitant coagulation (e.g., antiplatelet, NSAIDs) results in pharmacodynamic drug interactions that can increase the risk of bleeding and should be avoided as much as possible. After stopping fondaparinux, the anticoagulant effect will last up to 4 days and even longer in patients with low clearance [31].

Fondaparinux is not absorbed through the gastrointestinal mucosa, so it must be given parenterally. Subcutaneous administration showed rapid absorption and complete absorption with 100% bioavailability. The peak plasma concentration is reached about 2–3 h after subcutaneous administration. A stable state is achieved after 3–4 doses of administering fondaparinux once a day [25].

Fondaparinux is highly protein bound and cannot be distributed to tissues without binding to proteins. The volume of distribution is 7–11 L, which is close to blood volume. Fondaparinux does not undergo metabolism in the liver and is not susceptible to the pharmacokinetics of drug interactions with the cytochrome P450 isoenzyme system substrate [25].

Reduced bonding with macrophages and endothelial cells increases the half-life of plasma fondaparinux compared to UFH and LMWH. Elimination of fondaparinux is influenced by several patient parameters, including kidney function, age, and low body weight. These factors must be evaluated regularly, because they can block the use of fondaparinux or require increased monitoring for signs and symptoms of drug accumulation [25].

5.4 Ultralow molecular heparin

Therapy using LMWH provides clear pharmacokinetic advantages over UFH, so LMWH has become the standard of care for prevention and treatment of venous thromboembolism (VTE) in patients with and without cancer. The development of the ULMWH drug is based on the theory that, because of the much higher ratio of anti-Xa and anti-IIa activity, ULMWH will be associated with similar or better antithrombotic efficacy from the efficacy achieved by LMWH products but with lower bleeding and HIT risks. ULMWH has a molecular weight of <4000 Da and an increase in anti-factor Xa activity compared to LMWH. There is only one ULMWH marketed outside the United States (bemiparin), and another, RO-14, is currently in clinical development [32].

5.4.1 Pharmacokinetics and pharmacodynamics

Bemiparin was approved for once-daily use of subcutaneous VTE primary prophylaxis in medical patients and patients undergoing general or orthopedic surgery and for prophylaxis in patients with deep vein thrombosis (DVT). Bemiparin originates from alkaline depolymerization and UFH fractionation from pig intestinal mucosa. Pharmacokinetic studies in healthy volunteers given bemiparin showed an increase in anti-factor Xa activity depending on the dose given [32].

6. Heparin therapy monitoring

Treatment using UFH requires routine monitoring to see its functional activity due to the high variation in plasma concentrations and functional activities after fixed doses in each patient. This is due to several reasons, including AT levels in plasma that are different in each patient, UFH elimination with two mechanisms that also differ in each individual, and neutralization and bonding of heparin with various activated plasma proteins and platelets. It is estimated that 10% of people are not sensitive to heparin. The nonlinear pharmacodynamics of UFH make it difficult to predict. Unfractionated heparin (UFH) is usually measured by APTT or activated coagulation time (for high levels of heparin), but this examination has a low sensitivity and is not standardized; besides, this examination is also not sensitive to the use of low-dose UFH as prophylaxis. The results also depend on the reagent and the instrument used. The reference value for this examination must be determined by each laboratory, so it is difficult to compare the results obtained from each laboratory [33].

Monitoring the therapy of coagulation UFH activity should be measured 6 h after bolus and 6 h after dose change. It takes 6 h for the heparin to reach a stable phase, so monitoring heparin therapy less than 6 h after administration gives the wrong results for determining the dose. Protamine titration is the gold standard for heparin monitoring, but this examination is not widely available and expensive, so it is only used for research [34].

Unlike UFH, LMWH has a more stable pharmacokinetics, and its bioavailability reaches 100% at any dose with subcutaneous administration. The maximum LMWH concentration in plasma is directly proportional to the LMWH dose, and many experts believe that routine coagulation monitoring during therapy is not necessary because the clinical dose of LMWH can be corrected based solely on the patient's body weight. In a healthy population after a fixed dose of LMWH, it turns out that heparin concentration varies and only partially correlates with the patient's body weight. More precisely correction needs to be done in some cases (e.g., low or high BMI; critical condition; kidney failure (creatinine clearance <30 ml/min); when changing anticoagulants; age (children or elderly >75 years); and pregnancy) [35].

Anti-Xa activity measurement is the most widely used examination for LMWH therapy management. This examination has a high sensitivity (lower limit of determination using chromogenic substrate is <0.03 anti-Xa IU/mL). This method is not a method of global coagulation examination because it only measures the concentration of one factor (Xa) but does not react with AT deficiency or changes in concentration from other factors that influence patient hemostasis. This method is difficult to predict thrombosis or bleeding. Until now there is still no universal and reliable method for monitoring heparin properly [30].

6.1 Activated partial thromboplastin time (APTT)

The APTT examination is currently used by most laboratories for monitoring UFH therapy. This examination uses plasma citrate from the patient and is measured based on clot formation. Phospholipids and activators are added to platelet-poor plasma (PPP) patients and then incubated. Calcium is added and then the clotting time is measured. This examination has several advantages, fast, inexpensive, and widely available, but this does not directly measure the level of heparin. Many APTT reagents are available, and each reagent has a varied response to heparin therapy, and besides that several physiological factors can influence the results of this examination [36].

The clinical condition of patients can also affect the results of APTT, but it does not correlate with the presence of bleeding or thrombosis. The most frequent cases are patients receiving vitamin K antagonist therapy. Patients with international normalized ratio (INR) of more than 1.3 because warfarin therapy can also affect APTT results in heparin monitoring. Other cases that also affected were patients with antiphospholipid antibodies, which could affect clotting tests. Coagulation factor deficiencies, such as in patients with liver disease, or consumptive coagulopathy in disseminated intravascular coagulopathy (DIC) will affect APTT results. These conditions cause heparin anticoagulation activity not to be measured properly [36].

The conditions mentioned above can prolong the APTT results and result in underdose anticoagulant doses. Factor VIII and fibrinogen are the most frequent causes and can significantly extend or shorten the APTT baseline. Patients with acute disease are also known to have a deficiency in antithrombin. This condition can lead to excessive anticoagulation when using APTT for monitoring [36].

Preanalytic variables also play a role in the APTT response in monitoring heparin. The wrong APTT results can be due to improper sampling, and less samples also make too much citrate concentration in the tube. Underdose therapy causes a high risk of thrombosis [37].

Basu et al. [38] conducted a study on patients with venous thromboembolism who received heparin therapy and found the risk of recurrent thromboembolism associated with the APTT ratio which did not reach 1.5–2.5 times the normal value. This ratio is used as a standard for therapeutic ranges. Based on this study, the authors mention that the ratio is equivalent to levels of heparin 0.2–0.4 U/mL based on protamine titration and is equivalent to anti-Xa levels of 0.3–0.7 U/mL. The range of anti-Xa levels is higher because of heparin clearance. Smaller heparin molecules are cleared more slowly, so LMWH has a stronger inhibitory effect on factor Xa than thrombin. Examinations that measure anti-factor Xa activity, such as anti-Xa examination, will detect higher levels than examinations that measure antithrombin activity, such as protamine titration, which utilizes thrombin time [30].

Other studies evaluated the upper limit of anti-Xa examinations related to the incidence of bleeding. This study produced anti-Xa levels of more than 0.74–0.88 U/mL related to the incidence of bleeding complications [30]. The use of the APTT standard ratio for the range of heparin therapy is difficult to apply because the response of each APTT reagent to heparin is different. Researchers from the joint study found that APTT corresponds to a concentration of heparin 0.2–0.4 U/mL with protamine titration, based on the APTT reagent used. APTT reagents from other laboratories showed different sensitivity to heparin, and a ratio of 1.5–2.5 times the normal value did not correlate with the concentration of heparin in the therapeutic range. Various types of laboratories and reagents can produce an APTT ratio of 1.6–3.7 times the normal value, which is equivalent to a level of heparin 0.3 U/mL to a ratio of 2.4–6.2 times the normal value equivalent to the level of heparin 0.7 U/mL with anti-Xa [39].

6.2 Anti-Xa activity assay

Variations in results were also obtained for each anti-Xa examination if compared with protamine titration as a reference but far smaller compared to APTT. The therapeutic range for this examination will remain to be 0.3–0.7 U/mL, although with different machines and reagents. In contrast to APTT, anti-Xa results are not affected by poor sampling, also are not affected by factor VIII or fibrinogen, and are not affected by deficiency factors in patients with liver disease and consumptive coagulopathy [30].

Anti-Xa assay is not a test of factor X activity or factor X level antigen. This examination is also called an anti-factor Xa test or a functional test of heparin. The principle of this examination is to monitor indirect factor Xa inhibitors, such as LMWH and fondaparinux, or direct factor Xa inhibitor drugs such as rivaroxaban. These anticoagulants require monitoring in certain patient populations and in certain clinical settings. Each anticoagulant requires its own anti-X curve, and this must be done by each laboratory [37].

Anti-Xa activity assay uses the chromogenic method. The known factor Xa is added to platelet-poor plasma, wherein there is heparin. Heparin strengthens the inhibition of antithrombin to factor Xa, and the uninhibited factor Xa chromogenic substrate is added. This process produces color detected by a spectrophotometer and directly proportional to the level of factor Xa. The amount of color correlates with the level of heparin in the plasma with the correct heparin curve [36].

Like other tests, the anti-Xa assay is imperfect, with the chromogenic method; this examination will be affected by the conditions of the hemolysis, jaundice, and lipemic samples, which will affect the ability of the machine to measure and distinguish chromogenic reactions. Anti-Xa reagents which are not added with antithrombin will make false low heparin concentrations in the condition of patients with severe antithrombin deficiency, but there can be a misdiagnosis of antithrombin deficiency if antithrombin is added. Viewed from the laboratory side, anti-Xa assay is considered expensive and needs special attention in the process [36].

6.3 Protamine titration

Protamine is a small protein, rich in arginine, and positively charged, has a similarity to histones, and is involved in folding and stabilizing DNA in sperm heads. Protamine can neutralize the effects of heparin through electrostatic bonds between cation arginine groups from protamine and heparin anions with a ratio of 1:1. This results in a neutral protamine-heparin aggregate which can be seen in the form of a white suspense formed in a few seconds. Binding of heparin by protamine will release the AT-heparin complex, resulting in AT activity returning to its original state [40].

Protamine titration is the gold standard for measuring UFH concentrations in plasma. The results of this examination are quite promising, but it is still not considered a good examination in terms of clinical management of UFH because it is still not automatic. UFH clinical trials determined that heparin concentrations of 0.2–0.4 U/mL with protamine titration were equivalent to APTT lengthening 1.5–2.5 times the normal values, providing safe UFH levels and good patient outcomes [41].

The principle of this examination is to measure thrombin clotting time (TCT), which is the time required for clot formation after the addition of thrombin to plasma. The presence of UFH in plasma will result in TCT prolongation depending on the dose used. Protamine competed in binding to UFH, and the results of protamine titration measurements showed the amount of protamine needed to restore TCT to baseline [42].

This method is neither expensive nor difficult, but because it is done manually, the workload is quite heavy. The results given by this examination are very dependent on two important factors, the operator that works and the origin of thrombin. Protamine titration measurements depend on the operator when identifying clot formation in the test tube, so efforts to standardize this are difficult. The reproducibility of results can be achieved by limiting operators who work on checks and equating perceptions between operators about the process of forming clots and when the test is certain to be completed.

First time this method was found, thrombin used came from rabbits or young cattle. Its concentration is determined by identifying the amount of thrombin which results in TCT 18–20 s. At present the thrombin used is from humans, so it can increase the specificity of this test. Thrombin originating from humans has different interactions with plasma patients than thrombin from rabbits and young cattle. Thrombin originating from humans also needs to be determined by calculating the amount of thrombin needed to achieve TCT 18–20 s. Each laboratory must determine the concentration of thrombin that is needed based on thrombin available in each lab [41].

UFH therapy is optimal if the levels are 0.2–0.4 IU/mL based on protamine titration. Recommendations from the American College of Chest Physicians (ACCP) suggest that the APTT target for the UFH therapy range is equivalent to 0.2–0.4 IU/mL with protamine titration of 0.35–0.7 IU/mL with anti-Xa assay [23].

This method is carried out at room temperature, plasma samples and protamine solutions that have been titrated at each concentration, and thrombin stored in ice until it is transferred to the test tube. First take a normal plasma, and leave it at room temperature for 30 s. Then the titration solution is added, and thrombin is then calculated when the clot is formed. The time obtained will be used as TCT baseline. Assay was repeated using a sample of patients with different protamine concentrations starting from the highest concentration first (0.9 IU/mL). After finding the smallest concentration that still provides TCT baseline, this result illustrates the level of heparin in the blood [41].

6.4 Thrombodynamics

A new examination for the coagulation function, thrombodynamics (TD), is examined under different circumstances. This TD measures the level of clot formation. Coagulation is triggered on the surface of an activator which is bound to a space and extends to the plasma layer. The scattered beam increases in the area formed by the clot, so clot formation and time needed can be measured. This method is considered most able to mimic the coagulation process that occurs in vivo compared to other examinations. This examination is very sensitive to the conditions of either hypocoagulation or hypercoagulation. **Figure 5** shows the

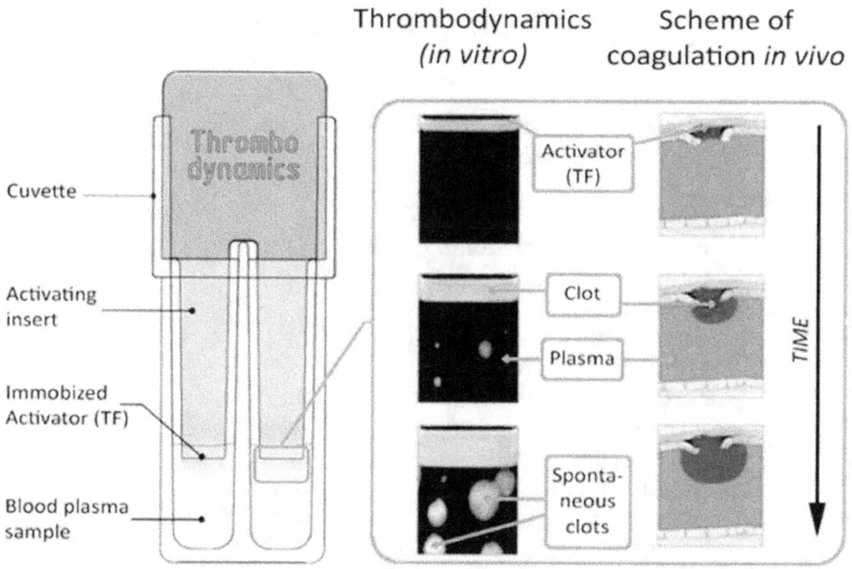

Figure 5.
Examination of thrombodynamics simulates the in vivo coagulation process. (a) Plastic cuvette schemes and activators that have been added for TD measurements. (b) Photos of the sequence of clot growth from spontaneous activator in vitro and clot in a portion of the sample. (c) Schematic image of clot growth from damage to blood vessel walls in vivo [44].

test tube scheme used in TD examination and the formation of clots and compared with the process of clot in vivo [43].

Clot formation curve depends on several parameters obtained: Tlag (time of formation of clot); Vi (initial speed of formation of clots) and V (speed of formation of clots) in clot formation (slope of clot formation curve versus time at 2–6 min and 15–25 min from the initial formation of clots for Vi and V); and CS (clot size 30 min after the coagulation process is activated). Other important parameters that are also measured are the maximum optical density of the formed clot (D) which shows the quality of the clot and the time required for the appearance of spontaneous clot (Tsp). The last two parameters have important clinical values because spontaneous clot (which grows not from activators on the surface) is only found in serious hypercoagulability states [44].

Heparin anticoagulants form complexes with ATIII and inhibit factors II, X, and IX. Research by Sinauridze et al. measure Tlag, Vi, and V parameters in post hip surgery patients who get heparin. The result is only Vi and V have significant different results, whereas Tlag has results that are not much different before and after heparin is given [44].

7. Conclusion

Heparin monitoring is needed to achieve an adequate dose. Laboratory tests for heparin monitoring include APTT examinations especially for UFH, anti-FXa activity assays especially for LMWH, protamine titration especially for UFH, and thrombodynamic tests that better reflect in vivo conditions.

Abbreviations

ACCP	American College of Chest Physicians
APC	activated protein C
APTT	activated partial thromboplastin time
AT	antithrombin
C1inh	C1 inhibitor
DIC	disseminated intravascular coagulopathy
DNA	deoxyribonucleic acid
GAG	glycosaminoglycans
HC II	heparin cofactor II
HIT	heparin-induced thrombocytopenia
INR	international normalized ratio
IV	intravenous
LMWH	low molecular weight heparin
NSAID	nonsteroid anti-inflammatory drug
PCI	percutaneous coronary intervention
PCI	protein C inhibitor
PF4	platelet factor 4
PN-1	protein nexin-1
PPP	platelet-poor plasma
SC	subcutaneous
Serpin	serine protease inhibitor
SFNG	symbol nomenclature for glycans
STEMI	ST-segment elevation myocardial infarction
TCT	thrombin clotting time
TD	thrombodynamics

TFPI	tissue factor pathway inhibitor
UFH	unfractionated heparin
ULMWH	ultralow molecular weight heparin
VTE	venous thromboembolism

Nomenclature

Symbols

CS	clot size at 30th minute of the measurement (μm)
D	clot density, it is an optical parameter, which is equal to intensity of light scattering from a fibrin clot (au)
Tlag	time between contact of plasma sample with activator and start of clot growth. Tlag characterizes the initiation phase of blood coagulation (min)
Tsp	time of spontaneous clot formation in plasma sample volume, which had no initial contact with activating insert. Spontaneous clotting is induced by circulating activators, active coagulation factors, and microparticles (min)
V	average rate of clot growth. The parameter characterizing the propagation phase of blood coagulation (μm/min)
Vi	initial rate, it characterizes the initiation phase of clot growth (μm/min)

Superscript

a	in normal renal function

Author details

Yetti Hernaningsih* and Ersa Bayung Maulidan
Department of Clinical Pathology, Faculty of Medicine, Dr. Soetomo General Academic Hospital, Universitas Airlangga, Surabaya, Indonesia

*Address all correspondence to: yettihernaningsih@gmail.com

References

[1] Arbit E, Goldberg M, Gomez-orellana I, Majuru S. Oral heparin: Status review. Thrombosis Journal. 2006;**4**:6

[2] Zmuda K, Ascp MT, Neofotistos D, Ts C. Effects of unfractionated heparin, low-molecular-weight heparin, and heparinoid on thromboelastographic assay of blood coagulation. Coagulation and Transfusion Medicine. 2000;**113**:725-731

[3] Oduah EI, Linhardt RJ, Sharfstein ST. Heparin: Past, present, and future. Pharmateuticals. 2016;**9**(38):1-12

[4] Garcia DA, Baglin TP, Weitz JI, Michel M. Parenteral Anticoagulants: Antithrombotic Therapy and Prevention of Thrombosis, 9th ed: American College of Chest Physicians Evidence-Based Clinical Practice Guidelines. Chest. 2012;**141**(June)

[5] Gray E, Mulloy B, Barrowcliffe TW. Heparin and low-molecular-weight heparin. Thrombosis and Haemostasis. 2008;**99**:807-818

[6] Schwarb H, Tsakiris DA. New direct oral anticoagulants (DOAC) and their use today. Dentistry Journal. 2016;**4**(1):5

[7] Huntington JA. Serpin structure, function and dysfunction. Journal of Thrombosis and Haemostasis. 2011;**9**:26-34

[8] Versteeg HH, Heemskerk JWM, Levi M, Reitsma PH. New fundamentals in coagulation. Physiological Reviews. 2013;**93**(January):327-358

[9] Ellery PER, Adams MJ, Rcpa F. Tissue factor pathway inhibitor: Then and now. Seminars in Thrombosis and Hemostasis. 2014;**40**(November):881-886

[10] Huntington JA. Mechanisms of glycosaminoglycan activation of the serpins in hemostasis. Journal of Thrombosis and Haemostasis. 2003;**1**:1535-1549

[11] Mulloy B, Hogwood J, Gray E, Lever R, Page CP. Pharmacology of heparin and related drugs. Pharmacological Reviews. 2016;**68**(January):76-141

[12] Izaguirre G, Aguila S, Qi L, Swanson R, Roth R, Rezaie AR, et al. Conformational activation of antithrombin by heparin involves an altered exosite interaction with protease. Journal of Biological Chemistry. 2014;**289**(49):34049-34064

[13] Wiebe EM, Stafford AR, Fredenburgh JC, Weitz JI. Mechanism of catalysis of inhibition of factor IXa by antithrombin in the presence of heparin or pentasaccharide. Journal of Biological Chemistry. 2003;**278**(37):35767-35774

[14] Mosier PD, Krishnasamy C, Kellogg GE, Desai UR. On the specificity of heparin/heparan sulfate binding to proteins. Anion-binding sites on antithrombin and thrombin are fundamentally different. PLoS One. 2012;**7**(11):1-12

[15] Tollefsen DM. Vascular Dermatan Sulfate and Heparin Cofactor II. I. Biochemistry of HCII [Internet], Progress in Molecular Biology and Translational Science: Glycosaminoglycans in Development, Health and Disease. Vol. 93. Elsevier Inc.; 2010. 351-372 p. DOI: 10.1016/S1877-1173(10)93015-9

[16] Huntington JA. Natural inhibitors of thrombin. Thrombosis and Haemostasis. 2014;**111**(January):583-589

[17] Huntington JA. Thrombin inhibition by the serpins. Journal of Thrombosis and Haemostasis. 2013;**11**:254-264

[18] Van Walderveen MC, Berry LR, Chan AKC. Effect of covalent antithrombin-heparin on activated protein C inactivation by protein C inhibitor. Journal of Biochemistry. 2010;**148**(2):255-260

[19] Bouton M, Boulaftali Y, Richard B, Arocas V, Jandrot-perrus M, Dc W, et al. Emerging role of serpinE2/protease nexin-1 in hemostasis and vascular biology. Blood. 2012;**119**(January):2452-2457

[20] Boulaftali Y, Ho-tin-noe B, Pena A, Loyau S, Venisse L, Richard B, et al. Platelet protease nexin-1, a serpin that strongly influences fibrinolysis and thrombolysis. Circulation. 2011;**123**(March):1326-1334

[21] Yang L, Ding Q, Huang X, Olson ST, Rezaie AR. Characterization of the heparin-binding site of the protein Z-dependent protease inhibitor. Biochemistry. 2012;**51**(March):4078-4085

[22] Konings J, Cugno M, Suffritti C, Cate H, Cicardi M, Govers-JWP. Ongoing contact activation in patients with hereditary angioedema. PLoS One. 2013;**8**(8):1-9

[23] Cm JH, Raschke R. Heparin and low-molecular-weight heparin the seventh ACCP conference on antithrombotic and thrombolytic. Chest. 2004;**126**(3):188S-203S. DOI: 10.1378/chest.126.3_suppl.188S

[24] Malloy RJ, Rimsans J, Rhoten M, Sylvester K, Fanikos J. Unfractionated heparin and low-molecularweight heparin. In: Anticoagulation Therapy. Springer; 2018. pp. 31-57

[25] Weitz DS, Weitz JI, Parenteral FÁ. Update on heparin: What do we need to know? Journal of Thrombosis and Thrombolysis. 2010;**29**(November):199-207

[26] Alquwaizani M, Buckley L, Adams C, Fanikos J. Anticoagulants: A review of the pharmacology, dosing, and complications. Current Emergency & Hospital Medicine Reports. 2013;**1**(April):83-97

[27] Gehrie E, Laposata M. Test of the month test of the month: The chromogenic antifactor Xa assay. American Journal of Hematology. 2012;**87**(October):194-196

[28] Zalpour A, Kroll MH, Afshar-kharghan V, Yusuf SW, Escalante C, Hematology B, et al. Role of factor Xa inhibitors in cancer-associated thrombosis: Any new data? Advances in Hematology. 2011;**2011**(July)

[29] Weitz JI. Factor Xa or thrombin: Is thrombin a better target? Journal of Thrombosis and Haemostasis. 2007;**5**(March):65-67

[30] Lehman CM, Frank EL. Laboratory monitoring of heparin therapy: Partial thromboplastin time or anti-Xa assay? Lab Medicine. 2009;**40**(1):47-51

[31] Bergqvist D. Review of fondaparinux sodium injection for the prevention of venous thromboembolism in patients undergoing surgery. Vascular Health and Risk Management. 2006;**2**(4):365-370

[32] Walenga JM, Lyman GH. Evolution of heparin anticoagulants to ultra-low-molecular-weight heparins: A review of pharmacologic and clinical differences and applications in patients with cancer. Critical Reviews in Oncology/Hematology. 2013;**88**(1):1-18. DOI: 10.1016/j.critrevonc.2013.06.007

[33] Takemoto CM, Streiff MB, Shermock KM, Kraus PS, Chen J, Jani J, et al. Activated partial thromboplastin time and anti-Xa measurements in heparin monitoring. Biochemical basis for discordance. Coagulation and transfusion Medicine. 2013;**139**:450-456

[34] Kinnard T. Anti-Xa Assay for Heparin Monitoring [Internet]. Mayo Clinic Laboratory; 2016. pp. 1-12. Available from: https://news.mayocliniclabs.com/2016/08/01/anti-xa-assay-for-heparin-monitoring-hot-topic/

[35] Fareed J, Hoppensteadt D, Walenga J, Iqbal O, Ma Q. Pharmacodynamic and pharmacokinetic properties of enoxaparin. Implications for Clinical Practice. Clinical Pharmacokinetics. 2003;**42**(12):1043-1057

[36] Bates SM, Weitz JI. Coagulation assays. Circulation. 2015;**112**(May):53-61

[37] Vandiver JW, Pharm D, Vondracek TG, Pharm D. Antifactor Xa levels versus activated partial thromboplastin time for monitoring unfractionated heparin. Pharmacotherapy. 2012;**32**(6):546-558

[38] Basu D, Gallus A, Hirsh J, Gade J. A prospective study if the value of monitoring heparin treatment with the activated partial tromboplastin time. New England Journal of Medicine. 1972;**287**(7):324-327

[39] Hirsh J, Anand SS, Halperin JL, Fuster V. A statement for healthcare professionals. Circulation. 2001;**103**(February):2994-3018

[40] Boer C, Meesters MI, Veerhoek D, Vonk ABA. Anticoagulant and side-effects of protamine in cardiac surgery. British Journal of Anaesthesia. 2018;**14**(January). DOI: 10.1016/j.bja.2018.01.023

[41] Walker JM. Haemostasis Methods and Protocols. Australia MP Department of PU of MPV, editor. Humana Press; 2013

[42] Bain BJ, Bates I, Laffan MA. Dacie and Lewis Practical Haematology. Elsevier Inc; 2017. 599 p

[43] Soshitova NP, Karamzin SS, Balandina AN, Fadeeva OA, Kretchetova AV, Galstian GM. Predicting prothrombotic tendencies in sepsis using spatial clot growth dynamics. Blood Coagulation & Fibrinolysis. 2012;**23**(February):498-507

[44] Sinauridze EI, Vuimo TA, Tarandovskiy ID, Ovsepyan RA, Surov SS, Korotina NG, et al. Thrombodynamics, a new global coagulation test: Measurement of heparin efficiency. Talanta. 2018;**180**(December):282-291

Section 3

Anticoagulant Therapy: Patients Overview and Perspectives

Chapter 5

Knowledge, Adherence, and Quality of Life among Warfarin Therapy Users

Laila Mahmoud Ali Matalqah

Abstract

Patient knowledge and understanding of the therapy are an important factor in treatment success. Multiple factors were identified to cause a treatment failure such as side effects of the medications, rejection of the diagnosis by patients, lack of patient understanding about their medication, noncompliance, and the cost of medication. In addition, improvements in patient medication counseling and education may help in prevention of many adverse drug interactions, drug-drug or food-drug interactions, in turn enhancing medication adherence which depends basically on a patient's acceptance of the information about the health threat itself. For these reasons, an evaluation of patients' knowledge of medicine and its use may help screen for problems in therapy and improve therapeutic outcomes. The results of this evaluation may also be used to educate providers about areas of potential problems in which they may be able to influence change.

Keywords: warfarin, knowledge, adherence, quality of life

1. Anticoagulation therapy

Coumarins have been used clinically since the 1950s and are likely the most widely studied medicines currently in clinical use [1, 2]. Anticoagulation therapy with warfarin has been a standard clinical practice to prevent ischemic stroke in patients associated with atrial fibrillation (AF) [3–6]. A meta-analysis demonstrates that adjusted-dose warfarin reduces stroke risk by 64% when compared to placebo, which is corresponding to an absolute annual risk reduction in all strokes of 2.7%, while antiplatelet agents reduce stroke risk by 22% [7]. In the ACTIVE W trial, anticoagulation therapy had a relative risk reduction of all strokes by 40% when compared to the combination of clopidogrel and aspirin, with no difference in bleeding events between both treatments [8]. Furthermore, anticoagulants may reduce the risk of death rate in AF patients by 38% [9], so about 70–80% patients with AF are suitable for the long-term use of warfarin [10, 11].

However, it increases the risk for major bleeding. Clinical studies revealed that the risk of intracranial hemorrhage, the most common type of bleeding, is as great as that of thromboembolic events warfarin is used to prevent [12, 13].

Therefore, the optimal use of warfarin for atrial fibrillation requires precise assessment of established risk factors of bleeding, such as advanced age, hypertension, stroke, alcoholism, and malignancy [14]. In addition, rigorous reporting of warfarin-associated bleeding is warranted, as patients who bleed often discontinue treatment, which put them at a higher risk of thromboembolism [15, 16].

1.1 Warfarin pharmacodynamics

Warfarin is a drug derived from 4-hydroxycoumarin group and acts by inhibiting vitamin K epoxide reductase, an enzyme which recycles vitamin K into its reduced form (**Figure 1**). Reduced vitamin K is responsible for carboxylation of the specific blood clotting factors II (prothrombin), VII, IX, and X as well as anticoagulant factor protein C and protein S [18–20]. Thus warfarin is not a direct antagonist of vitamin K but rather acts by depletion of reduced vitamin K in tissues.

As shown in **Figure 2**, inhibition of the reduction of vitamin K results in a reduction in the conversion of fibrinogen to fibrin which in turn reduces clot formation.

1.2 Warfarin pharmacokinetics

Warfarin is a racemic mixture of two optically active isomers, the R and S enantiomers [18]. Warfarin is highly water soluble and rapidly absorbed from the gastrointestinal tract and has high bioavailability [22, 23]. The bioavailability of warfarin is more than 95% [24, 25], and some reports had applied 100% bioavailability when developing models [26, 27].

Warfarin reaches maximal blood concentrations about 1.5 hours after oral administration [22, 28]. The plasma half-life of racemic warfarin mixture is 36–42 hours [29], and this means that it takes 5–7 days to reach steady state since warfarin is started or when the dosage is adjusted.

The antithrombotic effect of vitamin K anticoagulants has conventionally been attributed to their anticoagulant effect, which in turn is mediated by the reduction of the four vitamin K-dependent coagulation factors (II, VII, IX, and X). The vitamin K-dependent clotting factors have varying half-lives: 6 hours for factor VII, 24 hours for factor IX, 36 hours for factor X, and 60–72 hours for factor II (prothrombin). Thus, the anticoagulant effect (reduce coagulation of blood, prolonging the clotting time) develops in 2 days, whereas an antithrombotic effect (reduce formation of blood clots (thrombi)) of warfarin requires 6 days of treatment [30].

Numerous environmental factors such as drugs, diet, and various disease states were identified to affect warfarin by altering its kinetics and dynamics [31]. Drugs such as cholestyramine can reduce the absorption of warfarin, thus reducing its anticoagulant effect. R-warfarin is metabolized primarily by CYP1A2 and CYP3A4, while S-warfarin is metabolized primarily by CYP2C9 [32]. Potential warfarin drug interactions could occur with a concomitant administration of medicines that are metabolized by these P450s, and as a consequence, a number of metabolic medicine interactions have been reported for warfarin. For example, drugs such as cimetidine, amiodarone, and omeprazole potentiate the anticoagulant effect of warfarin by inhibiting its metabolism, whereas some drugs like barbiturates, rifampin, azathioprine, and carbamazepine inhibit the anticoagulant effect by enhancing its clearance [33]. In addition, long-term alcohol consumption has a similar potential to increase the clearance of warfarin [34].

Aspirin [35] and nonsteroidal anti-inflammatory drugs (NSAIDs) increase the risk of warfarin-associated bleeding by inhibiting platelet function [36].

1.3 Dietary vitamin K

As the action of warfarin is modified by vitamin K, a variable dietary intake of vitamin K may alter the extent of the anticoagulation effect. An increased intake of

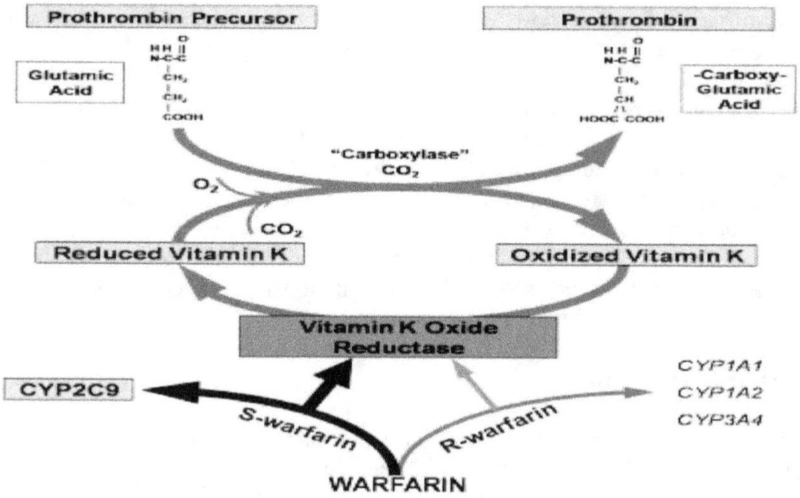

Figure 1.
Mechanism of action of warfarin [17].

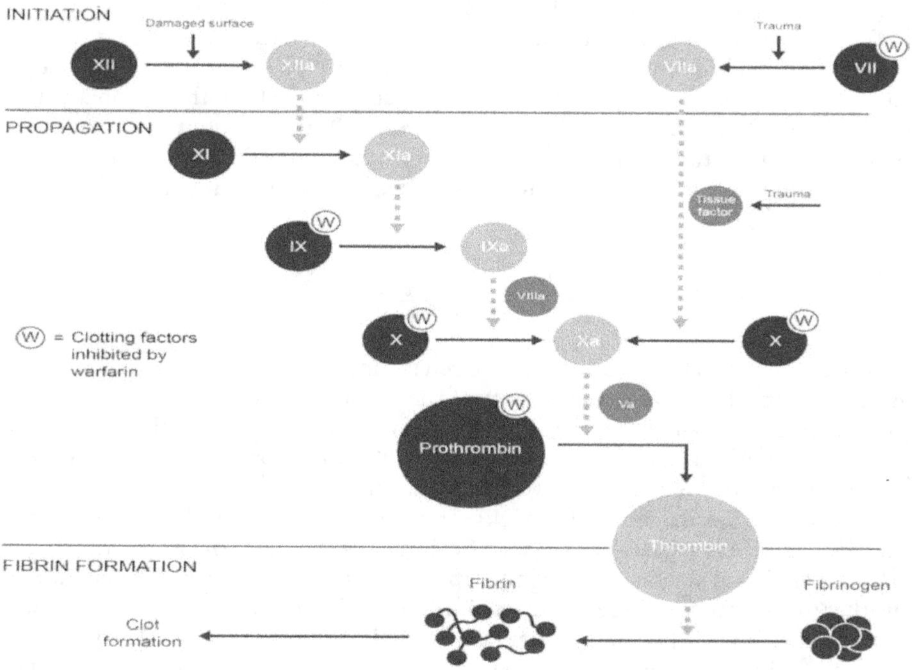

Figure 2.
Warfarin's effects on the clotting cascade [21].

dietary vitamin K (foods high in vitamin K include leafy green vegetables (cooked and raw), broccoli, brussels sprouts, cabbage, pickled cucumber, asparagus, kiwifruit, okra, green beans, and salad greens like lettuce) or vitamin K-containing supplements will increase the production of functional coagulation factors depending on vitamin K which is sufficient to reduce the anticoagulant response to warfarin [37]. Furthermore, patients with poor dietary intake of vitamin K often have a less stable control of anticoagulation [38]. It has been suggested to provide these unstable anticoagulated patients (with poor vitamin K intake) with oral vitamin K supplementation. However, unrecognized intake of such can lead to warfarin resistance [37].

The drug-grapefruit juice interaction enhances plasma concentration (C_{max}) of orally concomitantly administered drugs. This interaction has been reported with 40 pharmaceutical products, including the vitamin K antagonist [39]. Grapefruit can affect the metabolism of a variety of medications through the cytochrome P450 enzyme system located in the small intestine and liver. The enzymes that are affected are 3A4, 1A2, and 2A6. The (R) enantiomer of warfarin is metabolized by CYP1A2 and CYP3A4, which could contribute to this theoretical interaction of warfarin with grapefruit [40].

1.4 Warfarin monitoring

The relation between blood clotting and coumarin derivatives was established by Dam and Doisy who shared the Nobel Prize in 1943 for their work [41, 42]. Warfarin has a narrow therapeutic index in which effectiveness and safety are a tight balance between stroke risk and bleeding risk; hence, careful dose titration and monitoring are required.

The prothrombin time (PT) test is the most common test used to monitor vitamin K anticoagulant therapy [43]. The normal prothrombin time is 12–14 seconds [44]. As PT monitoring of warfarin treatment is not standardized when expressed in seconds, a calibration model which was adopted in 1982 is now used to standardize reporting by converting the PT ratio measured with the local thromboplastin into an international normalized ratio (INR) [45]. INR is calculated by raising the prothrombin time ratio (PT; the patient's prothrombin time divided by a reference normal prothrombin time to the power of international sensitivity index (ISI)) as follows (Eq. (1)):

$$INR = \left(\frac{\text{Patient PT}}{\text{Mean normal PT}}\right)^{ISI} \tag{1}$$

where ISI relates the sensitivity of a given thromboplastin (a tissue factor used as a reagent in PT test) to the sensitivity of the World Health Organization's first primary international reference preparation of thromboplastin, which was assigned an ISI of 1.0 [46]. Each manufacturer assigns an ISI value for any tissue factor they manufacture which is usually between 1.0 and 2.0.

Instead of a specific value of the INR target, a therapeutic window is utilized as the recommended target range for specific diagnosis, e.g., in atrial fibrillation the clinical benefits of warfarin are highly dependent on maintaining the INR within the therapeutic range of between 2 and 3, while mechanical heart valve replacement often requires a slightly higher target range of INR (2.5–4.0) [47–50]. As shown in **Figure 3**, INRs below this range increase the risk of stroke, while INR values above 3 or 4 are associated with increased bleeding rate [51].

Further quality assessment of the treatment involves calculation of time spent in the therapeutic range (TTR). In Rosendaal method, the difference between two consecutive INR readings, which was within the target range, was divided by the total difference between them [52].

1.5 Warfarin-related adverse drug events

The most common side effect from over-anticoagulation is bleeding from any anatomical site. There are many risk factors that increase the risk of hemorrhage

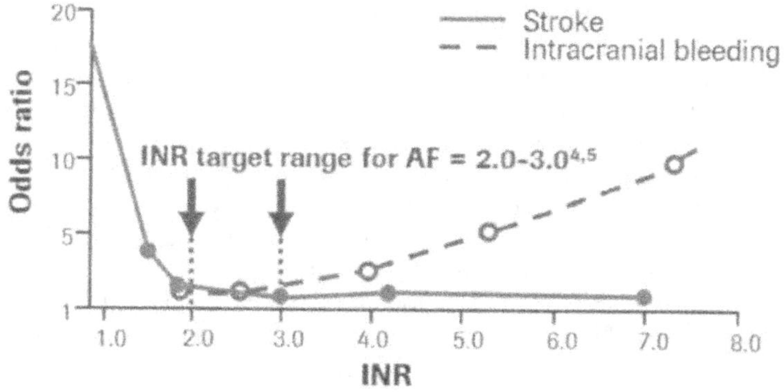

Figure 3.
Maintaining INR in the therapeutic range is crucial to prevent strokes and avoid bleeding [51].

in patients on oral anticoagulant therapy, such as increasing age (≥60); previous stroke; comorbidities, i.e., diabetes mellitus; recent myocardial infarction; anemia (defined as hematocrit <30%); the presence of malignancy; concomitant; antiplatelet usage; uncontrolled hypertension; liver/renal failure; and previous gastrointestinal bleed [53].

The most feared hemorrhagic complication of anticoagulants is the intracranial hemorrhage (ICH) which accounts for approximately 90% of deaths from warfarin-associated hemorrhage and for the majority of disability among survivors [54]. Nonetheless, ICH rates in clinical trials conducted in AF patients on oral anticoagulant therapy are small, reported to be between 0.3 and 0.6% per year [55], and the absolute increase in major extracranial hemorrhages is even smaller, at ≤0.3% per year [56]. The risk of ICH associated with warfarin use was twice that of aspirin, but the absolute risk was small at 0.2% per year [7].

Other than hemorrhage, other important side effects of warfarin are acute thrombotic complications, such as skin necrosis and limb gangrene [57, 58].

2. Patients' knowledge about warfarin therapy

2.1 Factors impacting patient's knowledge about warfarin therapy

Evidence from the literatures suggests that patients' knowledge about their warfarin therapy is generally poor with many demographic and clinical factors influencing their level of knowledge [2, 59–74].

IN the USA, a 52-item questionnaire related to the knowledge of warfarin was administered to 100 patients with atrial fibrillation in a face-to-face interview with a dietitian [69]. The survey questions were compiled based on five categories: general warfarin knowledge, compliance, drug interactions, herbal or vitamin interactions, and diet. For the total population, the average percentage of correct responses was 36%. The average score by category was 64% (general knowledge), 71% (compliance), 17% (drug interactions), 7% (herbal or vitamin interactions), and 23% (diet). Results from the former study suggested that in general, patients on warfarin, especially those at highest risk of stroke, had a poor understanding of their medication.

In Germany, in a study aimed to investigate the patients' knowledge on anticoagulants and the patient characteristics associated with low knowledge, an 8-item multiple-choice test was developed and distributed to 59 anticoagulated medical inpatients of a German university hospital [66]. The scoring range was 0–8 points (each correct answer giving 1 point). The average knowledge was 55% with the most often wrong answers about questions regarding drug-drug and drug-food interactions. The former study revealed no significant correlation between the total test score and any of the patient characteristics.

McCabe and colleagues [68] described the self-management knowledge and behaviors of patients with recently detected AF. One hundred subjects were interviewed by telephone to assess knowledge after 2-week hospitalization. They found a knowledge deficit related to the purpose of medication and complications of warfarin. The knowledge deficits were greater in older subjects and in subjects with less formal education. The patients aged between 65 and 74 years had knowledge scores of 26.6 (out of a possible 50), as compared to 19.1 for those aged between 75 and 94 years ($P = 0.001$); this may be due to cognition disorders. Despite knowledge deficits among the patients, they were high adherent to taking medication and anticoagulation monitoring.

In England, a pilot study to examine patient's knowledge and perceptions of AF and their anticoagulant treatment before and after a brief educational intervention was conducted [67]. Thirty-three patients completed the baseline interview; by then, they were given an information booklet which explained about AF, treatment options and their benefits/risks, and what the INR is and what factors may affect it. They were reassessed to their knowledge and perceptions of AF in a follow-up assessment session. Out of 33 (35.5%) patients that completed the follow-up assessment, 52% were aware about anticoagulants preventing blood clots, which increased to 70% post-intervention. However, few patients were aware of the benefit of stroke prevention associated with anticoagulants. The intervention significantly improved patient's knowledge of the target INR range and factors that may affect INR levels ($P = 0.001$ and $P = 0.014$, respectively); however, it had little effect on increasing awareness of the bleeding risks associated with anticoagulants.

To measure patient's knowledge about warfarin and to identify factors related to higher level of knowledge, Hu et al. [64] conducted a telephone survey among 100 patients with mitral valve replacement (MVR) using a validated 20-item questionnaire. They found that about 61% of participants had insufficient knowledge of warfarin therapy (score $\leq 80\%$). Among all variables studied, age was negatively related to warfarin knowledge scores, while family incomes greater than US$25,000, education greater than grade 8, and being employed significantly related to higher warfarin knowledge scores ($P < 0.05$). However, gender and ethnicity were not related to warfarin knowledge scores.

Besides all literatures mentioned above, the knowledge of warfarin therapy was tested in a sample of 122 patients attending at the warfarin clinic using 9 questions with a maximum score of 1.0 [71]. They found the level of knowledge was generally poor with more obvious knowledge deficient about the possible consequences of under- or over-anticoagulation, drugs that might interact with warfarin, and management of a missed dose. In their study, they found that increasing age negatively impacts upon knowledge about warfarin therapy. The mean warfarin knowledge scores declined with advancing age; <65-year-olds scored 0.47; 65–74-year-olds scored 0.44; and >75-year-olds scored 0.39. Other sociodemographic factors such as lower family income, limited health literacy, unemployment status, and lower education levels appeared to negatively influence patients' knowledge. However, they did find a weak but positive correlation between patients' knowledge of warfarin therapy and the number of INR values that were within the target range (Correlation coefficient r 0.20, $P = 0.024$).

Roche-Nagle et al. [2] evaluated the patient perception of anticoagulation risks, tablet recognition skills, and complications of warfarin therapy in 150 patients attending the anticoagulation clinic. Majority of the patients (n = 125, 83%) were able to identify the 1 mg tablet correctly, 105 (70%) identified the 3 mg tablet, and 98 (65%) identified the 5 mg tablet correctly. In addition, about 60% were aware about the potential complications from over- and underdosage with warfarin; however, only 33 (22%) were unaware that restrictions on alcohol use are required when taking warfarin. This study suggested that patient knowledge regarding anticoagulation therapy is not optimal, and consequently, a significant group may be at risk from serious complications because of this inadequate knowledge.

To investigate whether the knowledge and perceptions of antithrombotic therapy differ between ethnic groups in the UK, Nadar et al. [75] conducted a cross-sectional questionnaire survey among 180 patients attending anticoagulation clinic (135 white European, 29 Indo-Asian, and 16 Afro-Caribbean). The average knowledge score among all participants was 5.5 out of 9, with no significant differences between all ethnic groups. However, this study highlighted the gaps in the knowledge of patients from ethnic minorities and suggested that these groups should receive a special attention in the provision of information. Moreover, they have identified age as a negative factor of warfarin knowledge with the lowest score among patients older than 61 years.

In a historical cohort with questionnaires to 242 patients discharged from hospital, identified from hospital pharmacy records as being prescribed warfarin frequency of testing and levels of INR within 6 months of discharge, the level of INR aimed at by GP, complication rates, and patient knowledge about anticoagulation were measured [72]. Only 27% of all patients answered more than 8 out of 10 questions correctly. In this study, higher education level was identified as a predictor of high knowledge, but there was no relationship between the knowledge level and the INR control.

In Qatar, a cross-sectional survey using a 20-question questionnaire was delivered to 140 patients who were taking warfarin for at least 2 months [76]. Out of 12 questions about warfarin knowledge, 10 questions were derived from the Oral Anticoagulation Knowledge (OAK) test that was developed by Zeolla et al. [77]. The OAK questions covered the topics on warfarin drug interaction; interpretation of INR value, food, and vitamin K; effect of missing a dose; and when to seek a medical attention. In this study, the satisfactory level was considered answering 10 out of 12 questions (≥75%). They found that 79 patients (56%) had a satisfactory level of knowledge. The lowest score was in the knowledge of management of missing a dose and drug-drug interaction.

Another study using the OAK test was conducted in Jordan among 117 patients using warfarin, who were selected randomly [78]. They found that the majority (64%) of respondents can distinguish between different strengths of warfarin tablets by color. However, a deficit in knowledge was obvious in the areas of vitamin K and drug interactions with warfarin, skipping dose management, and PT/INR test. It was suggested that including clinical pharmacist services in the anticoagulation clinics may result in the improvement of patients' knowledge toward warfarin use and PT/INR test.

In a study sought to determine the level of knowledge and to what extent patients adhere to OAC therapy, Van Damme et al. [79] developed a questionnaire comprising 10 multiple-choice questions, including 2 questions about each of the 5 knowledge domains: (1) general information about the functioning of the medication, (2) possible side effects, (3) interactions with food, (4) drug interactions, and (5) lifestyle. For each question, four possible answers were given, one of which was correct. In this cross-sectional study which included 57 patients, the median total score on the knowledge questionnaire was 7 on a scale of 0–10 with only 9 patients (15.7%) answering more than 8 questions correctly. They found that the participants had moderate to poor knowledge regarding the kinds of medication that can be taken in case of headaches, the sports to be avoided, what to do when a dose of medication is missed, symptoms related to uncontrolled level of medication in the blood, the effect of alcohol in blood-thinning, and the influence of certain vitamins on the medications.

Finally, another study aimed to collect information on six items of anticoagulation counseling (mode of action of warfarin, adverse effects of over or under anticoagulation, drugs to avoid, action if bleeding or bruising occurs, and alcohol consumption) from 70 consecutive patients on anticoagulant therapy [74]. They found that most patients reported are being clearly advised on five of the six items, but their knowledge about anticoagulation was generally poor. Few patients were able to correctly identify adverse conditions associated with poor control of anticoagulation: bleeding was identified by only 30 (60%), and bruising by 23 (56%), and only 7 (14%) could identify 3 or more self-prescribed agents which may interfere with warfarin.

2.2 Relation of patients' warfarin knowledge to their therapeutic outcomes

To date, there are important published literatures that highlight the level of patients' knowledge about warfarin and its relation to the therapeutic outcome, as well as education strategies and their impact on therapy outcomes. In these literatures, there is a general consensus that improved patient knowledge about warfarin therapy improving therapeutic outcomes [59, 66, 71, 80–82].

Kagansky et al. [80] have measured patient's knowledge about warfarin by a warfarin knowledge-testing questionnaire. The questionnaire was submitted to elderly patients (n = 323) to assess their knowledge and impression on the quality of the relevant education that they received from the medical system on the following: risk of thromboembolic complications, prevention of thromboembolic complications by oral anticoagulation (OAC) therapy, the significance of OAC monitoring, and risk of bleeding. Among all participants, only 21.3% of the patients are satisfied about the education on OAC therapy that they received from the medical staff. In their study, patients with insufficient education on OAC therapy were more likely to increase major bleeding events (5.2 per 1000 patient-months) compared with no education (1.1 per 1000 patient-months). This study also showed that older patients with better knowledge about their warfarin therapy had 45% of their INR values within the therapeutic range than patients with poorer knowledge (35%); $P < 0.001$.

These findings were supported by another study [81] which reported that older patients (n = 125) who possessed a better understanding of warfarin therapy spent about 70% of the time within the therapeutic INR range than those with a poorer understanding (63%). The results of this latter study, however, were not statistically significant, reflecting the large amount of variability within each group and also possibly due to the limited number of patients included.

In Italy, Barcellona and colleagues [82] developed a questionnaire concentrated mainly on the patients' understanding of why they were taking oral anticoagulants, the mechanism of the therapy through its regular assumption, dietary behavior (vegetable intake), current diseases that did not require hospitalization, interactions with other drugs, and assumption of other drugs. It was administered to a group of 219 consecutive anticoagulated patients attending the thrombosis center. The percentage time spent in the therapeutic range was calculated using the INR Day Program by Rosendaal et al. [52]. The difference in time spent in the range between patients who knew why they were taking the oral anticoagulant and those who did not was statistically significant only in the older group (89% vs. 76%, $P = 0.04$).

In another study of Barcellona et al. [59], the time spent within the therapeutic range by patients taking oral anticoagulants was improved by two different, consecutive educational approaches on the crucial aspects of oral anticoagulant therapy. In this study, 240 patients were randomly allocated into three groups; a course that focused on the questions in the interview was given to the first group (n = 80); a brochure containing the correct answers to questions was given to the second (n = 81); nothing was provided for the third (n = 79). A significant difference was found in the TTR between the quarters preceding and following the interview with 13% increase in the mean TTR among all groups.

Not all studies have found a positive correlation between patient knowledge and outcomes of warfarin therapy. In a sample of 52 patients, knowledge of warfarin therapy was assessed with an 18-question multiple-choice test and associated with anticoagulation control [62]. The anticoagulation control was defined as the number of blood tests in the appropriate therapeutic range divided by the number of blood tests performed during the 60-day period. This study showed no significant association between knowledge or education and the proportion of INRs within the therapeutic range. Moreover, insufficient education on OAC as perceived by the patient or caregiver was one of the significant predictive factors for bleeding complications (OR 8.83).

In Fang et al.'s [83] study, health literacy was measured using the bilingual short-form Test of Functional Health Literacy in Adults (s-TOFHLA), dichotomized as "limited" (score 0–22) and "adequate" (score 23–36) among 179 anticoagulated English- or Spanish-speaking patients. INR control was assessed by calculating the time in therapeutic range for each patient using an adapted linear interpolation method [52], defined as the proportion of person-time within the target therapeutic range over the total person-time of follow-up. It was found that patients with limited health literacy were more likely to have incorrect answers to most questions addressing warfarin-related knowledge and numeracy with incorrect answers to questions about warfarin's mechanism of action, side effects, medication interactions, and frequency of monitoring, after adjusting for age, sex, ethnicity, education, cognitive impairment, and years on warfarin. However, limited health literacy was not significantly associated with TTR over the previous 12 months.

In the USA, another study aimed to explore the association between literacy and numeracy skills among patients on warfarin, and their anticoagulation control was conducted among 143 patients older than 50 years attending 2 anticoagulation clinics [84]. They found that The INR variability was higher among patients with lower literacy ($P = 0.009$) and lower numeracy skills ($P = 0.004$). The time in the range was similar among patients at different literacy levels ($P = 0.9$); however, patients with lower numeracy level spent more time above their therapeutic range ($P = 0.04$) and had a trend of less time spent in range ($P = 0.10$).

In Malaysia, two previous studies have been conducted to assess the patients' knowledge and relate their knowledge to INR control [85, 86]. Hasan et al. [85] assessed the anticoagulation knowledge and INR control among patients on warfarin. In this cross-sectional study, 156 randomly sampled patients were interviewed using a validated interviewer-administered questionnaire, and all patients' INR readings were recorded from 2008 to 2010. The authors found the average score of patients knowledge was 66.5% + 36.0% on how warfarin works, 42.9% + 44.9% for interaction between warfarin and alcohol, and 49.2% + 21.1% for adverse effects. Among all variable studied, they found a negative correlation between patients' knowledge and age ($P = 0.001$, $r = -0.293$) and a positive correlation between patients' knowledge and their education level ($P = 0.001$, $r = 0.365$). Furthermore, no significant correlation was found between patients' INR control and their knowledge on the mechanism of action of warfarin, the interaction between warfarin and alcohol, and the side effects of warfarin.

Another cross-sectional survey was conducted at the Warfarin Clinic of Hospital Teluk Intan, Malaysia, and tended to determine the factors that correlated with the patient's knowledge of warfarin therapy, the level of medication adherence, and INR control [86]. A total of 52 patients were interviewed with a mean ± SD age of 58.73 ± 9.55 years. Only 44.2% of patients knew about their medications, but the medication adherence was fairly good at 76.1%. The study showed that age, income level, level of education, and literacy in various languages were significantly associated with the patient's knowledge on warfarin therapy ($P < 0.05$). The study did not find any association between anticoagulation and the level of knowledge of anticoagulation. However, the major limitation of the former two studies is the limited sample size used.

It is also important to highlight that some of the aforementioned studies, regardless of their results, are limited by the use of a non-validated warfarin knowledge-testing instruments or questionnaire to evaluate patient knowledge [2, 66–69, 73–75, 86]. Validation indicates that the questionnaire has been thoroughly tested for content validity, measures of question difficulty, readability, and item/person reliability. Only after a knowledge assessment instrument has been validated can sound scientific conclusions be drawn from its results [87]. The appropriate psychometric methodology must be followed to ensure that an assessment measure is valid and reliable for testing the specific objectives or constructs. In theory, this process demonstrates that an instrument's results are accurate, consistent, reproducible, and stable over time [87–89].

To date, only two questionnaires measuring patient knowledge of warfarin therapy have been validated: the Oral Anticoagulation Knowledge test, created and validated by Zeolla et al. [77], and the Anticoagulation Knowledge Assessment (AKA) questionnaire, designed and validated by Briggs et al. [90].

In Zeolla et al. [77], the Oral Anticoagulation Knowledge, a new instrument, was developed by four nationally recognized anticoagulation experts to ensure content validity. The test was administered to 72 subjects on warfarin and 27 from a group of age-matched subjects not on warfarin to assess construct validity. Subgroups of warfarin subjects were retested approximately 2–3 months after initial testing to assess test-retest reliability. The OAK test was administered to 74 subjects taking warfarin and 27 age-matched subjects not on warfarin. In this study, subjects taking warfarin scored significantly higher than those not on warfarin (72% vs. 52%, respectively; $P < 0.001$), supporting the construct validity of the instrument. Test-retest reliability was acceptable, with a Pearson's correlation coefficient of 0.81, and the internal consistency reliability was 0.76. However, the association between the level of knowledge and clinical outcomes was not tested.

Another validated tool is the Anticoagulation Knowledge Assessment test, which was developed by Briggs et al. [90]. It is a 29-multiple-choice instrument that measures patient knowledge in 9 content areas, each worth 3.45 points. The validity of the instrument was assessed among 60 patients managed in two anticoagulation clinics who had received warfarin therapy for a mean of 28 months. The majority (80%) of patients who participated in the study had 12 or more years of education. The instrument was designed to be self-administered at a sixth grade reading level. Content validity of the instrument verified that the AKA instrument contains a variety of questions of varying levels of cognitive difficulty. However, the authors did not report whether they performed key reliability assessments (e.g., internal reliability or test-retest reliability); furthermore, they did not examine the relationship between patient's knowledge and the anticoagulation control.

In literature, Baker et al. [91] used the validated AKA questionnaire. Correctly answering 21 questions (72.4%) or more was needed for the determination of adequate knowledge of anticoagulation therapy (passing score). Interestingly, this cross-sectional study showed that 74% (n = 185) of patients receiving long-term warfarin therapy had achieved a pass rate. Statistically, no significant correlation between warfarin knowledge and INR control was found. These results may have been inflated as the questionnaire is a self-completed questionnaire at home and there is a possibility of assistance from others.

On the other hand, the impact of educational program in reducing the clinical adverse event rates was tested by a randomized trial [92]. They reported a decrease in the adverse event rates by threefold less in the educated group compared to the control group. This supports the significant and independent impact of the educational program on the reduction in risk of events (OR 0.25, 95% CI 0.1–0.7).

Similarly, other studies showed that patient knowledge has a positive effect in the clinical outcomes with the highest rate of major bleeding events among patients who had poor knowledge about warfarin [80, 93]. In Beyth et al.'s [93] study, there was a reduction in hospitalizations among patients receiving structured warfarin education compared to those in a control group (3 vs. 9 hospitalizations, respectively, out of a total of 12 hospitalizations; $P = 0.08$). Moreover, the time spent within the therapeutic range was higher in the educated group than in the control normal care group (56% vs. 32%; $P < 0.001$).

In summary, evidence from previous studies, such as Davis et al. [62] (n = 52), Fang et al. [83] (n = 139), Estrada et al. [84] (n = 143), Group TNAS [72] (n = 242), and Baker et al. [91] (n = 260) suggested no association between patients' warfarin knowledge and anticoagulation control. Some of the results of these latter studies, however, cannot be generalized because of their use of small sample sizes [62], number of variables relating to patient knowledge measured [62], and use of non-standardized data collection techniques [91].

The inverse relationship between the individual patient's level of knowledge about warfarin and the rate of adverse outcome events has been reported in other literatures [2, 68, 71, 80, 92].

3. Health-related quality of life of warfarin users

The term health-related quality of life (HRQoL) has been used when the concern of researchers is to investigate the influence of the disease and treatment on the quality of life of the individual [94]. This narrower concept has been used to avoid ambiguity between the definition of quality of life in the common sense and that used in clinical and medical trials.

Warfarin use is challenging [18], since it has a narrow therapeutic index; it interacts with other drugs, alcohol, and food [31, 95]; and the clinical response to it is affected by many factors such as patients' compliance and overall knowledge of therapy [74, 82]. Therefore, warfarin therapy requires a special care in order to control the desirable levels of blood coagulation and to prevent hemorrhagic and thromboembolic complications. Such care can lead to changes in the lifestyle of warfarin users since this involves changes in the dietary habits, the use of alcohol, and the performance of physical activity [96, 97], as well as the need to adhere strictly to the treatment regimen, the inconvenience of dosing adjustments, and the need for regular blood tests to monitor INR levels, together with the fear of complications such as the risk of minor or major bleeding and stroke [98]. All these changes caused by the use of anticoagulant treatment negatively affect the patient's

HRQoL. Perceived reduction in HRQoL is an important factor, which may influence the physician's prescription and patient's use of warfarin therapy.

To study the HRQoL of OAC users, authors have used different types of instruments. In a literature review regarding specific instruments available to evaluate the HRQoL of patients using OACs, the authors identified seven instruments [99]. In Brazil, a new specific instrument, the Duke Anticoagulation Satisfaction Scale (DASS), was developed by Samsa et al. [100] and recently validated by Pelegrino [101]. Some authors used a measurement of HRQoL obtained through the generic instrument such as the Medical Outcomes Survey 36-item Short Form (SF-36) [96, 100, 102, 103] and found that the more impaired HRQoL domains were physical aspects and vitality [96, 102], pain [100], physical functioning, and general health status [96].

In a cross-sectional study aimed to analyze the HRQoL and its relationship with gender, age, duration, and indication for the use of OAT, a total of 178 patients were interviewed, and the HRQoL was assessed through 8 domains of the SF-36 [104]. The means of the domains of the SF-36 ranged from 82 (social aspects) to 54.8 (physical aspects). In their study, the men had higher scores than the women in the majority of the domains of the SF-36, except for general health status. However, these differences were only significant in the domains, mental health, and pain. Elderly patients diagnosed with atrial fibrillation and with less than 1 year of medication use presented a worse HRQoL evaluation.

The HRQoL was also evaluated through a cross-sectional study with a sample composed of 72 patients with atrial fibrillation and mechanical heart valve at the anticoagulation outpatient unit of the Federal University of Bahia's University Hospital [105]. The patients were submitted to two quality of life evaluation questionnaires: SF-36 and DASS. The quality of life perception of the patients studied, based on both instruments, was positive regarding the treatment with OAC. The SF-36 presented an average score of 62.2 (±20.0). Among the SF-36 evaluated domains, the physical-emotional aspect was the most compromised one. The DASS presented an average score of 67.1 (±18.2), and the domain presenting a greater compromise was the one related to the treatment inconveniences. The authors identified many factors impacting patients' HRQoL; previous hemorrhagic event, comorbidities, drug interactions with medicines that increase the anticoagulant effect, lower education level in the SF-36, and younger age group influence a more negative perception of the QoL, whereas lower education level in the DASS and the duration of treatment for more than 1 year offer a more positive perception.

In a randomized, controlled trial including 333 atrial fibrillation patients using warfarin for stroke prevention, the impact of the long-term use of warfarin in their quality of life was assessed [97]. The results for their trial showed no significant differences between warfarin-treated and control patients on well-validated measures of functional status, well-being, and health perceptions. The mean score of health perceptions was 68.8 in the warfarin-treated group vs. 66.6 in the control group (scale of 0 to 100; 95% CI). In contrast, patients taking warfarin who had a bleeding episode had a significant decrease in health perceptions (−11.9; 95% CI). The authors concluded that warfarin therapy is not usually associated with a significant decrease in perceived health, unless a bleeding episode has occurred.

In an attempt to find the strategies to improve the HRQoL of patients undergoing anticoagulation therapy, a previous study found that patient self-management improves general treatment satisfaction and decreases patients' perception of treatment-related daily hassles, distress, and strain on their social network (Gadisseur et al., 2004). This is supported by other researchers who noted an improvement in many of treatment-related areas of QoL through patient self-management in comparison with routine anticoagulant care through family physicians [106, 107, 108].

4. Adherence toward warfarin

An assessment of warfarin adherence is important in improving patient's warfarin-taking behavior and INR control. Nonadherence includes not only a cessation of medication therapy but also taking the medication other than as prescribed (i.e., under-adherence, over-adherence, or not taking the dose at the prescribed time). Most studies reported medication adherence as a percentage of doses taken out of those prescribed over a specific period of time. While there is no general consensus on what constitutes adherence or nonadherence.

Nonadherence to OAC medication is generally problematic in practice. In a cohort study in the USA, 1005 patients with AF and taking warfarin are included, and there was a 32% reduction (from 65 to 44%) in the number of patients taking warfarin after 30 months [109].

Poor patient adherence to the prescribed drug regimen is often cited as an explanation for out-of-range INR measurements [110]. Despite this, there is little rigorous evidence of the level of adherence to warfarin, particularly among a broad spectrum of patients and anticoagulation practices. One reason for the lack of data on adherence to warfarin is the difficulty in measuring adherence [111].

In a prospective study of warfarin adherence, both under-adherence and over-adherence were measured among a sample of 145 patients at 3 anticoagulation clinics. The mean percentage of nonadherent days was 21.8% as measured by electronic medication event monitoring system (MEMS) [112].

In Singapore, another cross-sectional survey aimed to validate a patient-reported medication adherence measure, the MMAS-8, within a convenience sample of 151 patients taking warfarin [113]. It was found that respondents with higher MMAS-8 scores are more likely to have a higher percentage of INRs within the therapeutic range ($P = 0.01$), higher adherence to diet recommendations ($P = 0.02$), and less perceived difficulty in taking all medications ($P < 0.001$); they were also more likely to take warfarin at the same time every day ($P < 0.001$). This study showed that the 8-item MMAS has good validity and moderate reliability in patients taking warfarin.

In the International Normalized Ratio Adherence and Genetics (IN-RANGE) study of 111 adults taking warfarin, factors impacting patient adherence toward warfarin were studied [114]. It was found that demographic factors like education and occupation and psychosocial factors (such as lower levels of mental health functioning and poor cognitive functioning) are associated with nonadherence. Specifically, nonadherence was greater among those with educational levels beyond high school and those currently employed (compared with those unemployed and retired).

In a literature review by Brown et al. [115], many factors associated with OAC adherence among patients with AF were summarized as disease- and drug-related; patient knowledge, beliefs, and abilities; health system-related; economics; patient-physician relationship; and patient demographic, psychosocial, and personality traits.

In another review article that identified many factors associated with nonadherence in older adults, Murray et al. [116] developed a conceptual model of general medication adherence to improve adherence, assist in adherence research, and facilitate the development of multidimensional adherence improvement interventions. They concluded from an extensive literature search that older adults are at special risk due to the burden of multiple chronic diseases and age-related factors, such as cognitive impairment and other environmental and social factors.

To assess barriers to OAC medication use among patients with AF, a new questionnaire was developed by Ingelgård et al. [65]. The authors identified 41 barriers to warfarin use and classified them into 4 groups: patient medical characteristics, healthcare system factors, patient capability, and patient preference. On the other hand, Cohen et al. [117] summarized the factors that affect adherence to anticoagulation medication as factors related to disease (e.g., symptoms, long-term therapy, morbidities), drug (e.g., adverse events, duration, dose frequency and complexity, polypharmacy, cost), patient (e.g., lack of support, lack of disease knowledge, concerns, difficulty comprehending instructions, inability to adhere to restrictions), follow-up (e.g., shortage of time, costs associated with INR monitoring, patient unwilling to repeat testing, delay in laboratory reporting), and health system (e.g., patient-doctor relationship, reimbursement, lack of proper facilities or experience to manage therapy).

Added to the previous literature, Arnsten et al. [118] found significant relationships between various demographic characteristics and adherence. Noncompliance patients were more likely than warfarin-adherent patients to be younger (mean age 53.7 vs. 68.7 years), male, and nonwhite. Non-adherent patients were also more likely to report a lack of understanding or knowledge of the reason for taking warfarin and were also less likely to have a regular physician.

In Korea, a cross-sectional survey involving 204 patients aimed to identify factors affecting medication adherence and their relationships with anticoagulation control in Korean patients taking warfarin [119]. They found that 56 (27.5%) of 204 respondents were adherent. Their results showed that knowledge about warfarin exerts significant influence on medication adherence; however, medication adherence was not associated with good anticoagulation level as measured by INR.

The association between medication adherence and the clinical outcome of warfarin was also studied previously. In Davis et al. [62], adherence was found as one of the many factors that contribute to anticoagulation control. In this cross-sectional survey, the 4-item Morisky survey was used to assess self-reported adherence. The researchers found that adequate adherence was reported by 50% of patients and it was significantly associated with good anticoagulation control ($P = 0.01$) [120, 121].

In addition, this relationship between medication adherence and the clinical outcome of warfarin was also studied by Kimmel et al. [122]. In this prospective cohort study involving three coagulation clinics in Pennsylvania, 136 patients treated with warfarin for various indications (with a goal INR of 2–3), adherence to anticoagulation therapy was monitored using electronic MEMS medication bottle caps. The authors found patients who fail to adhere to warfarin therapy as prescribed are more likely to experience problems with anticoagulation control. Patients who missed >20% of bottle openings are two times more likely to have under-coagulation (adjusted OR 2.10). On the other hand, a significant effect on INR with over-adherence was also demonstrated; patients who had >10% extra pill bottle openings had a statistically significant increase in over-coagulation (adjusted OR 1.73). Furthermore, the authors estimated that poor patient adherence to medications is responsible for more than 53% of all hospital admissions.

In contrast, another cross-sectional study studied the relationship between adherence and other factors with the INR stability [123]. Among all patients, 90% ($n = 156$) had high and medium adherence, and 117 (75%) had INR stability up to 50% and 39 (25%) $\geq$ 75%. It was found that factors like adherence, age, level of education, socioeconomic level, interaction with other drugs, comorbidities, and vitamin K intake did not influence INR stability. However, longer anticoagulation time and drug cost were the factors related to the anticoagulation stability.

In studies among patients with diagnoses other than AF and on anticoagulation therapy, other psychosocial factors associated with poorer adherence were identified. These factors include depressive symptoms, pessimism, and a perceived lack of social support [111, 124, 125].

5. Factors impacting anticoagulation control

A retrospective cross-sectional study was conducted in community clinics in Israel aimed to assess the level of anticoagulation control achieved in patients with AF and to explore patient factors that influence the anticoagulation control [126]. The univariate and multivariate analyses were performed to explore the association of patient variables with anticoagulation control. They found that the mean TTR was 48.6% with about two-thirds of patients had poor anticoagulation control, as evidenced by TTR of <60%. Poor control was significantly associated with female sex, advancing age, and comorbid conditions. Heart failure was found to be an independent predictor of poor control (OR: 1.63).

A different cohort methodology was applied for assessing the likelihood of poor INR control among AF patients [127]. They used linear regression analysis to detect clinical factors associated with TTR and binary logistic regression to evaluate the predictive factors for different cut-off values of TTR. They explored various variables as independent predictors of poor TTR: female gender, age <50 years, ethnic minority status, smoking, more than two comorbidities, and being treated with a beta blocker, verapamil, or, inversely, amiodarone use.

Author details

Laila Mahmoud Ali Matalqah
Department of Basic Medical Sciences, Faculty of Medicine, Yarmouk University, Irbid, Jordan

*Address all correspondence to: laila.m@yu.edu.jo

References

[1] Link KP. The discovery of dicumarol and its sequels. Circulation. 1959;**19**:97-107

[2] Roche-Nagle G, Chambers F, Nanra J, Bouchier-Hayes D, Young S. Evaluation of patient knowledge regarding oral anticoagulants. Ireland Medical Journal. 2003;**96**(7):211-213

[3] Connolly SJ, Laupacis A, Gent M, Roberts RS, Cairns JA, Joyner C. Canadian atrial fibrillation anticoagulation study. Journal of American College of Cardiology. 1991;**18**:349-355

[4] Ezekowitz MD, Bridgers SL, James KE, Carliner NH, Colling CL, Gornick CC, et al. Warfarin in the prevention of stroke associated with nonrheumatic atrial fibrillation. New England Journal of Medicine. 1992;**327**:1406-1412

[5] Katritsis DG, Gersh BJ, Camm AJ. Anticoagulation in atrial fibrillation—Current concepts. Arrhythmia & Electrophysiology Review. 2015;**4.2**:100-107. PMC. Web. 15 Jan. 2018

[6] Xu J, Luc JG, Phan K. Atrial fibrillation: Review of current treatment strategies. Journal of Thoracic Disease. 2016;**8**(9):E886

[7] Hart RG, Pearce LA, Aguilar MI. Meta-analysis: Antithrombotic therapy to prevent stroke in patients who have nonvalvular atrial fibrillation. Annals of Internal Medicine. 2007;**146**:857-867

[8] Connolly S, Pogue J, Hart R, Pfeffer M, Hohnloser S, Chrolavicius S, et al. Clopidogrel plus aspirin versus oral anticoagulation for atrial fibrillation in the Atrial fibrillation Clopidogrel Trial with Irbesartan for prevention of Vascular Events (ACTIVE W): A randomised controlled trial. Lancet. 2006;**367**:1903-1912

[9] Alpesh A. Oral anticoagulation to reduce risk of stroke in patients with atrial fibrillation: Current and future therapies. Clinical Interventions in Aging. 2013;**8**:75-84. DOI: 10.2147/CIA.S37818

[10] Darcy RF, Allan ER, Richard CB, Timothy ST. CYP2C9 genotype-dependent warfarin pharmacokinetics: Impact of CYP2C9 genotype on R- and S-warfarin and their oxidative metabolites. Journal of Clinical Pharmacology. 2017;**57**:382-393. DOI: 10.1002/jcph.813

[11] Liu XB, Huang HM, Yu JH, Gao GL, Feng LL, Xu Q, et al. Warfarin compared with aspirin for older Chinese patients with stable coronary heart diseases and atrial fibrillation complications. International Journal of Clinical Pharmacy and Therapeutics. 2014;**52**:454-459. DOI: 10.5414/CP201996

[12] Mittal MK, Rabinstein AA. Anticoagulation-related intracranial hemorrhages. Current Atherosclerosis Reports. 2012;**14**(4):351-359. DOI: 10.1007/s11883-012-0258-8 [Review]

[13] Senoo K, Lane D, Lip GY. Stroke and bleeding risk in atrial fibrillation. Korean Circulation Journal. 2014;**44**(5):281-290. DOI: 10.4070/kcj.2014.44.5.281

[14] Hughes M, Lip GY. Risk factors for anticoagulation-related bleeding complications in patients with atrial fibrillation: A systematic review guideline development group for the NICE national clinical guideline for management of atrial fibrillation in primary and secondary care. Quarterly Journal of Medicine. 2007;**100**(10):599-607

[15] Healey JS, Oldgren J, Ezekowitz M, et al. Occurrence of death and

stroke in patients in 47 countries 1 year after presenting with atrial fibrillation: A cohort study. Lancet. 2016;**388**:1161-1169

[16] Steinberg BA, Piccini JP. Anticoagulation in atrial fibrillation. British Medical Journal. 2014;**348**:g2116. DOI: 10.1136/bmj.g2116

[17] Pharmaceutical Information. 2013. Available from: http://www.pharmainfo.net/pettho/blog/warfarin-part-i

[18] Ansell J, Hirsh J, Hylek E, Jacobson A, Crowther M, Palareti G, et al. Pharmacology and management of the vitamin K antagonists. Chest. 2008;**133**:160-198

[19] Malhotra OP, Nesheim ME, Mann KG. The kinetics of activation of normal and gamma-carboxyglutamic acid-deficient prothrombins. The Journal of Biological Chemistry. 1985;**260**:279-287

[20] Friedman PA, Rosenberg RD, Hauschka PV, Fitz-James A. A spectrum of partially carboxylated prothrombins in the plasmas of coumarin-treated patients. Biochimica et Biophysica Acta. 1977;**494**:271-276

[21] The use of dabigatran in general practice: A cautious approach is recommended. Best Practice Journal. 2011. Available from: http://www.bpac.org.nz/magazine/2011/september/dabigatran.asp [Accessed: March 2013]

[22] Breckenridge AM. Oral anticoagulant drugs: Pharmacokinetic aspects. Seminars in Hematology. 1978;**15**:19-26

[23] O'Reilly RA. Vitamin K and other oral anticoagulant drugs. Annual Review of Medicine. 1976;**27**:245-261

[24] Juno Y, Rengarajan B, Yoo BK. Self-nanoemulsifying drug delivery system of lutein: Physicochemical properties and effect bioavailability of warfarin. Biomolecules & Therapeutics. 2013;**21**:173-179. DOI: 10.4062/biomolther.2013.011

[25] Mark K, Dennis G, Veronica M. Warfarin bioavailability with feeding tubes and enteral formula. Journal of Parenteral and Enteral Nutrition. 2010;**34**:300-304. DOI: 10.1177/0148607109337257

[26] Hamberg AK, Dahl ML, Barban M, Scordo MG, Wadelius M, Pengo V, et al. A PK-PD model for predicting impact of age, CYP2C9 and VKORC1 genotype on individualization of warfarin therapy. Clinical Pharmacology and Therapeutics. 2007;**81**:529-538. DOI: 10.1038/sj.clpt.610008

[27] Steven L, Sameh AZ, Ellen H, Ivan M, Andrea LJ, Panos D, et al. The population pharmacokinetics of R- and S-warfarin: Effect of genetic and clinical factors. British Journal of Clinical Pharmacology. 2011;**73**:66-76. DOI: 10.1111/j.1365-2125.2011.04051.x

[28] Kelly JG, O'Malley K. Clinical pharmacokinetics of oral anticoagulants. Clinical Pharmacokinetics. 1979;**4**:1-15

[29] O'Reilly RA. Warfarin metabolism and drug-drug interactions. In: Wessler S, Becker CG, Nemerson Y, editors. The New Dimensions of Warfarin Prophylaxis: Advances in Experimental Medicine and Biology. New York, NY: Plenum; 1986. pp. 205-212

[30] Zivelin A, Rao VM, Rapaport SI. Mechanism of the anticoagulant effect of warfarin as evaluated in rabbits by selective depression of individual procoagulant vitamin-K dependent clotting factors. Journal of Clinical Investigation. 1993;**92**:2131-2140

[31] Holbrook AM, Pereira JA, Labiris R, McDonald H, Douketis JD, Crowther M, et al. Systematic overview of warfarin

and its drug and food interactions. Archives of Internal Medicine. 2005;**165**:1095-1106

[32] Kaminsky LS, Zhang ZY. Human P450 metabolism of warfarin. Pharmacology and Therapeutic Journal. 1997;**73**(1):67-74

[33] Orme M, Breckenridge A. Enantiomers of warfarin and phenobarbital. New England Journal of Medicine. 1976;**295**:1482-1483

[34] O'Reilly RA. Lack of effect of fortified wine ingested during fasting and anticoagulant therapy. Archives of Internal Medicine. 1981;**141**:458-459

[35] Dale J, Myhre E, Loew D. Bleeding during acetylsalicylic acid and anticoagulant therapy in patients with reduced platelet reactivity after aortic valve replacement. American Heart Journal. 1980;**99**:746-751

[36] Battistella M, Mamdami MM, Juurlink DN, Rabeneck L, Laupacis A. Risk of upper gastrointestinal hemorrhage in warfarin users treated with nonselective NSAIDs or COX-2 inhibitors. Archives of Internal Medicine. 2005;**165**:189-192

[37] O'Reilly RA, Rytand D. Resistance to warfarin due to unrecognized vitamin K supplementation. New England Journal of Medicine. 1980;**303**:160-161

[38] Sconce E, Khan T, Mason J, Noble F, Wynne H, Kamali F. Patients with unstable control have a poorer dietary intake of vitamin K compared to patients with stable control of anticoagulation. Journal of Thrombosis & Homeostasis. 2005;**93**(5):872-875

[39] Saito M, Hirata-Koizumi M, Matsumoto M, Urano T, Hasegawa R. Undesirable effects of citrus juice on the pharmacokinetics of drugs. Drug Safety. 2005;**28**:677-694

[40] Sterling ES, Smith KM. What's the scoop with grapefruit? Orthopedics. 2005;**28**:31-34

[41] Dam H. The antihaemorrhagic vitamin of the chick. Biochemistry Journal. 1935;**29**:1273-1285

[42] MacCorquodale DW, Binkley SB, Thayer SA, Doisy EA. On the constitution of vitamin K1. Journal of American Chemistry & Society. 1939;**61**(7):1928-1929

[43] Quick AJ. The prothrombin time in haemophilia and in obstructive jaundice. The Journal of Biological Chemistry. 1935;**109**:73-74

[44] Hoffbrand AV. Essential Haematology. Oxford: Blackwell Science; 2002. p. 248

[45] Kirkwood TBL. Calibration of reference thromboplastins and standardisation of the prothrombin time ratio. Journal of Thrombosis & Haemostasis. 1983;**49**:238-244

[46] Dzung TL, Weibert RT, Sevilla BK, Donnelly KJ, Rapaport SI. The international normalized ratio (INR) for monitoring warfarin therapy: Reliability and relation to; other monitoring methods. Annual Internal Medicine. 1994;**120**:552-559

[47] Oake N, Jennings A, Forster AJ, Fergusson D, Doucette S, van Walraven C. Anticoagulation intensity and outcomes among patients prescribed oral anticoagulant therapy: A systematic review and meta-analysis. Canadian Medical Association Journal. 2008;**179**:235-244

[48] Odén A, Fahlén M, Hart RG. Optimal INR for prevention of stroke and death in atrial fibrillation: A critical appraisal. Thrombosis Research. 2006;**117**:493-499

[49] Hirsh J, Dalen JE, Anderson DR, Poller L, Bussey H, Ansell J, et al.

Oral anticoagulants: Mechanism of action, clinical effectiveness, and optimal therapeutic range. Chest. 2001;**119**(1):8S-21S

[50] Hylek EM, Skates SJ, Sheehan MA, Singer DE. An analysis of the lowest effective intensity of prophylactic anticoagulation for patients with nonrheumatic atrial fibrillation. New England Journal of Medicine. 1996;**335**:540-546

[51] Fuster V, Rydén LE, Cannom DS, Crijns HJ, Curtis AB, Ellenbogen KA, et al. ACC/AHA/ESC 2006 guidelines for the management of patients with atrial fibrillation. Circulation. 2006;**114**:e257-e354

[52] Rosendaal FR, Cannegieter SC, van der Meer FJM. A method to determine the optimal intensity of oral anticoagulant therapy. Journal of Thrombosis & Homeostasis. 1993;**69**:236-239

[53] Tay KH, Lane DA, Lip GY. Bleeding risks with combination of oral anticoagulation plus antiplatelet therapy: Is clopidogrel any safer than aspirin when combined with warfarin? Journal of Thrombosis & Haemostsis. 2008;**100**:955-957

[54] Fang MC, Go AS, Chang Y, Hylek EM, Henault LE, Jensvold NG, et al. Death and disability from warfarin-associated intracranialand extracranial haemorrhages. American Journal of Medicine. 2007;**120**:700-705

[55] Hart RG, Tonarelli SB, Pearce LA. Avoiding central nervous system bleeding during antithrombotic therapy: Recent data and ideas. Stroke. 2005;**36**:1588-1593

[56] Lip GY, Lim HS. Atrial fibrillation and stroke prevention. The Lancet Neurology. 2007;**6**(11):981-993

[57] Weinberg AC, Lieskovsky G, McGehee WG, Skinner DG. Warfarin necrosis of the skin and subcutaneous tissue of the male genitalia. Journal of Urology. 1983;**130**:352-354

[58] Verhagen H. Local hemorrhage and necrosis of the skin and underlying tissues at starting therapy with dicumarol or dicumacyl. Acta Medica Scandinavica. 1954;**148**:455-467

[59] Barcellona D, Contu P, Marongiu F. A "two-step" educational approach for patients taking oral anticoagulants does not improve therapy control. Journal of Thrombosis and Thrombolysis. 2006;**22**:185-190

[60] Cheah GM, Martens KH. Coumadin knowledge deficits: Do recently hospitalized patients know how to safely manage the medication? Home Healthcare Nurse. 2003;**21**(2):94-100

[61] Dantas GC, Thompson BV, Manson JA, Tracy CS, Upshur RE. Patients' perspectives on taking warfarin: Qualitative study in family practice. BMC Family Practice. 2004;**5**(1):15

[62] Davis NJ, Billett HH, Cohen HW, Arnsten JH. Impact of adherence, knowledge, and quality of life on anticoagulation control. Annals of Pharmacotherapy. 2005;**39**(4):632-636

[63] Engova D, Duggan C, MacCallum P, Bates I. Patients' understanding and perceptions of treatment as determinants of adherence to warfarin treatment. International Journal of Pharmacy Practice. 2002;**10**(suppl):R69

[64] Hu A, Chow C, Dao D, Errett L, Keith M. Factors influencing patient knowledge of warfarin therapy after mechanical heart valve replacement. Journal of Cardiovascular Nursing. 2006;**21**(3):169-175

[65] Ingelgård A, Hollowell J, Reddy P, Gold K, Tran K, Fitzmaurice D. What

are the barriers to warfarin use in atrial fibrillation? Development of a questionnaire. Journal of Thrombosis & Thrombolysis. 2006;**21**(3):257-265

[66] Jank S, Bertsche T, Herzog W, Haefeli WE. Patient knowledge on oral anticoagulants: Results of a questionnaire survey in Germany and comparison with the literature. International Journal of Pharmacology & Therapeutic. 2008;**46**(6):280-288

[67] Lane DA, Ponsford J, Shelley A, Sirpal A, Lip GYH. Patient knowledge and perceptions of atrial fibrillation and anticoagulant therapy: Effects of an educational intervention programme The West Birmingham Atrial Fibrillation Project. International Journal of Cardiology. 2006;**110**:354-358

[68] McCabe PJ, Schad S, Hampton A, Holland DE. Knowledge and self-management behaviors of patients with recently detected atrial fibrillation. Heart & Lung. 2008;**37**(2):79-90

[69] Smith MB, Christensen N, Wang S, Strohecker J, Day JD, Weiss JP, et al. Warfarin knowledge in patients with atrial fibrillation: Implications for safety, efficacy, and education strategies. Cardiology. 2010;**116**:61-69

[70] St-Louis L, Robichaud-Ekstrand S. Knowledge level and coping strategies according to coagulation levels in older persons with atrial fibrillation. Nursing & Health Science. 2003;**5**:67-75

[71] Tang EO, Lai CS, Lee KK, Wong RS, Cheng G, Chan TY. Relationship between patients' warfarin knowledge and anticoagulation control. Annual of Pharmacotherapy. 2003;**37**:34-39

[72] Group TNAS: The Newcastle Anticoagulation Study Group. Effectiveness of anticoagulation among patients discharged from hospital on warfarin. Medical Journal of Australia. 1998;**169**:243-246

[73] McCormack PM, Stinson JC, Hemeryck L, Feely J. Audit of an anticoagulant clinic: doctor and patient knowledge. Ireland Medicine Journal. 1997;**90**(5):192-193

[74] Taylor FC, Ramsay ME, Tan G, Gabbay J, Cohen H. Evaluation of patients knowledge about anticoagulation treatment. Quality in Health Care. 1994;**3**(2):7985

[75] Nadar S, Begum N, Kaur B, Sandhu S, Lip GY. Patients' understanding of anticoagulant therapy in a multiethnic population. Journal of Royal Society & Medicine. 2003;**96**:175-179

[76] Khudair IF, Hanssens YI. Evaluation of patients' knowledge on warfarin in outpatient anticoagulation clinics in a teaching hospital in Qatar. Saudi Medical Journal. 2010;**31**(6):672-677

[77] Zeolla MM, Brodeur MR, Dominelli A, Haines ST, Allie ND. Development and validation of an instrument to determine patient knowledge: The oral anticoagulation knowledge test. Annual of Pharmacotherapy. 2006;**40**(4):633-638

[78] Yassien AM, Khataybeh OY, Aleyadeh A, Al-kurdi NE, TA AL-S. Patients' experiences and knowledge about using coumarine and coagulation test. Zagaziq University Medical Journal. 2012;**18**(6):1118-1122

[79] Van Damme S, Van Deyk K, Budts W, Verhamme P, Moons P. Patient knowledge of and adherence to oral anticoagulation therapy after mechanical heart-valve replacement for congenital or acquired valve defects. Heart & Lung. 2011;**40**(2):139-146

[80] Kagansky N, Knobler H, Rimon E, Ozer Z, Levy S. Safety of anticoagulation therapy in

well-informed older patients. Archives of Internal Medicine. 2004;**164**:2044-2050

[81] Khan T, Kamali F, Kesteven P, Avery P, Wynne H. The value of education and self-monitoring in the management of warfarin therapy in older patients with unstable control of anticoagulation. British Journal of Haematology. 2004;**126**:557-564

[82] Barcellona D, Contu P, Marongiu F. Patient education and oral anticoagulation therapy. Hema. 2002;**87**(10):1081-1086

[83] Fang MC, Machtinger EL, Wang F, Schillinger D. Health literacy and anti- coagulation-related outcomes among patients taking warfarin. Journal of General Internal Medicine. 2006;**21**(8):841-846

[84] Estrada CA, Martin-Hryniewicz M, Peek BT, Collins C, Byrd JC. Literacy and numeracy skills and anticoagulation control. American Journal of Medical Science. 2004;**328**(2):88-93

[85] Hasan SS, Shamala R, Syed IA, Basariah N, Chong DW, Mei TK, et al. Factors affecting warfarin-related knowledge and INR control of patients attending physician- and pharmacist-managed anticoagulation clinics. Journal of Pharmacy Practice. 2011;**24**(5):485-493

[86] Yahaya AHM, Hassali MA, Awaisu A, Shafie AA. Factors associated with warfarin therapy knowledge and anticoagulation control among patients attending a warfarin clinic in Malaysia. Journal of Clinical Diagnostic Research. 2009;**3**:1663-1670

[87] Devellis RF. Scale Development: Theory and Applications. Newbury Park, CA: Sage Publications; 1991

[88] Kline P. A Handbook of Test Construction: Introduction to Psychometric Design. New York: Methuen & Co; 1986

[89] Streiner DL, Norman GR. Health Measurement Scales: A Practical Guide to Their Development and Use. New York: Oxford University Press; 1989

[90] Briggs AL, Jackson TR, Bruce S, Shapiro NL. The development and performance validation of a tool to assess patient anticoagulation knowledge. Research of Social & Administrative Pharmacy. 2005;**1**(1):40-59

[91] Baker WJ, Pierce KL, Ryals CA. INR goal attainment and oral anticoagulation knowledge of patients enrolled in an anticoagulation clinic in a veterans affairs medical Center. Journal of Managed Care Pharmacy. 2011;**17**(2):133-142

[92] Pernod G, Labarère J, Yver J, Gross R, Metlay JP, Christie JD, et al. EDUC'AVK: Reduction of oral anticoagulant-related adverse events after patient education: A prospective multicenter open randomized study. Journal of General Internal Medicine. 2008;**23**(9):1141-1146

[93] Beyth RJ, Quinn L, Landefeld CS. A multicomponent intervention to prevent major bleeding complications in older patients receiving warfarin: A randomized, controlled trial. Annals of Internal Medicine. 2000;**133**(9):687-695

[94] Fayers PM, Machin D. Scores and measurements: Validity, reliability and sensitivity. In: Quality of Life: Assessment, Analysis and Interpretation. 2nd ed. Chichester, England: John Wiley & Sons; 2007

[95] Greenblatt DJ, von Moltke LL. Interaction of warfarin with drugs, natural substances and foods. Journal of Clinical Pharmacology. 2005;**45**:127-132

[96] Casais P, Meschengieser SS, Sanchez-Luceros A, Lazzari MA. Patients' regarding oral anticoagulation therapy and its effect on quality of life. Current Medicine Research Opinions. 2005;**21**(7):1085-1090

[97] Lancaster TR, Singer DE, Sheehah MA, Oertel LB, Maraventano SW, Hughes RA, et al. The impact of long-term warfarin therapy on quality of life-evidence from a randomized trial. Archives of Internal Medicine. 1991;**151**:1944-1949

[98] McCahon D, Murray ET, Holder RL, Fitzmaurice DA. Does self-management of oral anticoagulation therapy improve quality of life and anxiety? Family Practice. 2011;**28**(2):134-140

[99] Wild D, Murray M, Shakespeare A, Reaney M, von Maltzahn R. Patient-reported treatment satisfaction measures for long-term anticoagulant therapy. Expert Review of Pharmacoeconomics & Outcomes Research. 2008;**8**:291-299

[100] Samsa G, Matchar DB, Dolor RJ, Wiklund I, Hedner E, Wygant G, et al. A new instrument for measuring anticoagulation-related quality of life: Development and preliminary validation. Health and Quality of Life Outcomes. 2004;**2**:22

[101] Pelegrino FM. Cultural Adaptation and Validation of Duke Instrument Anticoagulation Satisfaction Scale (DASS): Version for Brazilian in Use of Oral Anticoagulation. Ribeirão Preto: School of Nursing, University of São Paulo; 2009. p. 168

[102] Howes CJ, Reid MC, Brandt C, Ruo B, Yerkey MW, Prasad B, et al. Exercise tolerance and quality of life in elderly patients with chronic atrial fibrillation. Journal of Cardiovascular Pharmacology & Therapeutics. 2001;**6**(1):23-29

[103] Matchar DB, Jacobson AK, Edson RG, Lavori PW, Ansell JE, Ezekowitz MD, et al. The impact of patient self-testing of prothrombin time for managing anticoagulation: Rationale and design of VA cooperative study #481—The home INR study (THINRS). Journal of Thrombosis & Thrombolysis. 2005;**19**(3):163-172

[104] Corbi ISA, Dantas RAS, Pelegrino FM, Carvalho ARS. Health related quality of life of patients undergoing oral anticoagulation therapy. Revista Latino-Americana de Enfermagem. 2011;**19**(4):865-873

[105] Almeida GQ, Noblat LD, Passos LCS, Nascimento HF. Quality of life analysis of patients in chronic use of oral anticoagulant: An observational study. Health and Quality of Life Outcomes. 2011;**9**:91

[106] Cromheecke ME, Levi M, Colly LP, de Mol BJ, Prins MH, et al. Oral anticoagulation self-management and management by a specialist anticoagulation clinic: A randomised cross-over comparison. The Lancet. 2000;**356**(9224):97-102

[107] Kulinna W, Ney D, Wenzel T, Heene DL, Harenberg J. The effect of self-monitoring the INR on quality of anticoagulation and quality of life. Seminars in Thrombosis and Hemostasis. 1999;**25**:123-126

[108] Sawicki PT. A structured teaching and self-management program for patients receiving oral anticoagulation: A randomized controlled trial. Working Group for the Study of patient self-management of oral anticoagulation. Journal of American Medical Association. 1999;**281**:145-150

[109] Reynolds MR, Shah J, Essebag V, et al. Patterns and predictors of warfarin use in patients with new-onset atrial fibrillation from the FRACTAL registry.

American Journal of Cardiology. 2006;**97**(4):538-543

[110] Kutner M, Nixon G, Silverstone F. Physicians' attitudes toward oral anticoagulants and antiplatelet agents for stroke prevention In elderly parents with atrial fibrillation. Archives of Internal Medicine. 1991;**151**:1950-1953

[111] Osterberg L, Blaschke T. Adherence to medication. New England Journal of Medicine. 2005;**353**(5):487-497

[112] Parker CS, Chen Z, Price M, Gross R, Metlay JP, Christie JD, et al. Adherence to warfarin assessed by electronic pill caps, clinician assessment, and patient reports: Results from the IN-RANGE study. Journal of General Internal Medicine. 2007;**22**(9):1254-1259

[113] Wang Y, Kong MC, Ko T. Psychometric properties of the 8-item Morisky medication adherence scale in patients taking warfarin. Journal of Thrombosis &. Homeostasis. 2012;**108**(4):789-795

[114] Platt AB, Localio AR, Brensinger CM, Cruess DG, Christie JD, Gross R, et al. Risk factors for nonadherence to warfarin: Results from the IN-RANGE study. Pharmacoepidemiology & Drug Safety. 2008;**17**(9):853-860

[115] Brown TM, Siu KWD, Pladevall-Vila M, Sande S, Mordin M. Development of a conceptual model of adherence to oral anticoagulants to reduce risk of stroke in patients with atrial fibrillation. Journal of Managed Care Pharmacy. 2012;**18**(5):351-362

[116] Murray MD, Morrow DG, Weiner M, Clark DO, Tu W, Deer MM, et al. A conceptual framework to study medication adherence in older adults. American Journal of Geriatric Pharmacotherapy. 2004;**2**(1):36-43

[117] Cohen AT, Maillarde L, Yavin Y. Will a once-weekly anticoagulant for the treatment and secondary prevention of thromboembolism improve adherence? Journal of Thrombosis & Haemostasis. 2009;**101**(3):422-427

[118] Arnsten JH, Gelfand JM, Singer DE. Determinants of compliance with anticoagulation: A case-control study. American Journal of Medicine. 1997;**1103**(1):11-17

[119] Kim JH, Kim GS, Kim EJ, Park S, Chung N, Chu SH. Factors affecting medication adherence and anticoagulation control in Korean patients taking warfarin. Journal of Cardiovascular Nursing. 2011;**26**(6):466-474

[120] Morisky DE, Ang A, Krousel-Wood M, Ward H. Predictive validity of a medication adherence measure for hypertension control. Journal of Clinical Hypertension. 2008;**10**:348-354

[121] Morisky DE, Green LW, Levine DM. Concurrent and predictive validity of a self-reported measurement of medication adherence and long-term predictive validity of blood pressure control. Medical Care. 1986;**24**:67-74

[122] Kimmel SE, Chen Z, Price M, Parker CS, Metlay JP, Christie JD, et al. The influence of patient adherence on anticoagulation control with warfarin: Results from the International Normalized Ratio Adherence and Genetics (IN-RANGE) study. Archives of Internal Medicine. 2007;**167**:229-235

[123] Ávila CW, Aliti GB, Feijó MKF, Rabelo ER. Pharmacological adherence to Oral anticoagulant and factors that influence the international normalized ratio stability. Revista Latino-Americana de Enfermagem. 2011;**19**(1):18-25

[124] Cruess DG, Localio AR, Platt AB, Brensinger CM, Christie JD,

Gross R, et al. Patient attitudinal and behavioral factors associated with warfarin non-adherence at outpatient anticoagulation clinics. International Journal of Behavior Medicine. 2010;**17**(1):33-42

[125] Rieckmann N, Gerin W, Kronish IM, Burg MM, Chaplin WF, Kong G, et al. Course of depressive symptoms and medication adherence after acute coronary syndromes: An electronic medication monitoring study. Journal of American College of Cardiology. 2006;**248**(11):2218-2222

[126] Melamed OC, Horowitz G, Elhayany A, Vinker S. Quality of anticoagulation control among patients with atrial fibrillation. The American Journal of Managed Care. 2011;**17**(3):232-237

[127] Apostolakis S, Sullivan RM, Olshansky B, Lip GY. Factors affecting quality of anticoagulation control among patients with atrial fibrillation on warfarin: The SAMe-TT2R2 score. Chest. 2013;**144**(5):1555-1563

www.ingramcontent.com/pod-product-compliance
Lightning Source LLC
Chambersburg PA
CBHW081232100626
46462CB00006B/551
* 9 7 8 1 7 8 9 8 5 0 7 5 8 *